THIS IS ME!

MY JOURNEY WITH TURNER SYNDROME

THIS IS ME!

MY JOURNEY WITH TURNER SYNDROME

KELSEY SMITH

"Behind every successful woman is a tribe of successful women who have her back."

To my tribe (you all know who you are): This book is dedicated to you. Thank you for ALWAYS having my back. I'm beyond blessed to have such an amazing tribe surrounding me. I cannot imagine my life without you all.

Table of Contents

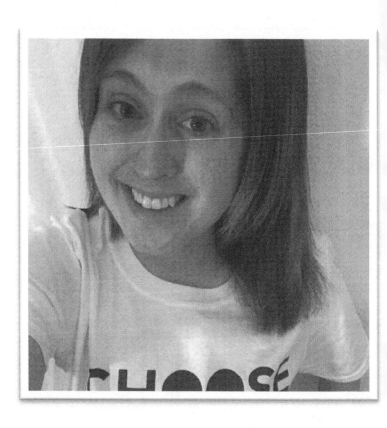

Introduction

Anne Frank once said, "How wonderful it is that nobody need wait a single moment before beginning to improve the world." This quote has resonated with me since the very first time I heard it. Personally, I believe there is so much truth to that saying. I believe that a person does have the ability to improve the world. Anne Frank's quote has been one that I try to live my life by. To be honest, that quote is the reason I wrote this book. I haven't always been ready to tell my story, but if the story I am about to tell can help even one person, then I am ready to tell it. It wasn't until recently, at the age of twenty-eight, that certain events in my life showed me I was ready. Once I knew I was ready to tell my story, I didn't want to wait a single moment longer. Now that I'm telling the story, I'm not going to hold anything back either.

Growing up, I never imagined that I would even entertain the idea of writing a book. Don't get me wrong. Writing is not something I dislike. Since I was nine, I have always kept a journal. I'll actually never forget the first journal I ever received. It was given to me by my mom and Great Aunt Joan for my ninth birthday. The journal had a hardcover and a picture of a large orange tabby cat on it. Once I received that gift, I constantly wanted to write. Writing in my journal is something that has always been relaxing and even de-stressing for me. Throughout the years, I have filled numerous journals with my writing. However, when it comes to writing, I never thought of myself as someone who would write a book.

I started to entertain the idea of writing a book when I thought that somehow my writing could have a positive impact. Telling the story that is about to unfold in this book is a big risk for me. It is a story that I did not openly tell many people until I was twenty-eight. One night though, I had the realization that maybe my story would help someone who is going through a situation similar to mine. It was at that moment that I promised myself to write it down. After all, this story is not something that I am ashamed of. It is about time that it is told.

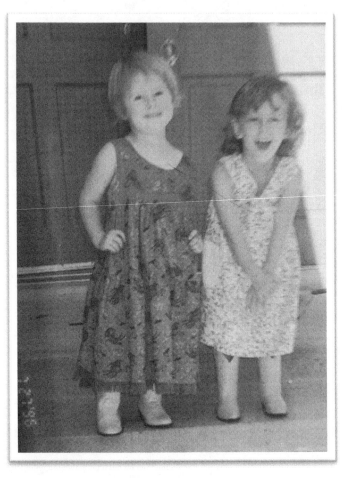

(My sister, Kaitlyn (on the left) and I standing outside our house in Denver, CO in 1996)

CHAPTER I

❖

Life in the 90s

To truly grasp and understand my story, some background information about me must first be told. I was born on January 10, 1990 in Englewood, Colorado. At the time, my parents, Marty and Sharon Smith, lived in Denver, and I was their first child. My father worked for the Denver Sheriff's Department, and my mother was the Vice President of APG Security. I like to joke and say that I am a "product of law enforcement" since both my parents have been involved in the field. My parents made Denver, Colorado home because as an employee of the Denver Sheriff's Department, my father had to live there.

On October 1, 1992, my life changed, and I was no longer an only child. It was on that day that my sister, Kaitlyn, made her entrance into the world. Growing up, my relationship with my sister had its ups and downs. I think anyone with a sibling can relate to that. In the end though, I was always happy to have a sister. I vaguely remember the day that my mother brought my sister home from the hospital. Since that day, my sister has always made life interesting (in a good way). Thousands of miles may separate my sister and me now, but we have remained amazing friends since that day in October 1992. I couldn't imagine my life without a sibling. Kaitlyn may be my sister by chance, but we grew into amazing friends by choice.

We lived in our house in Denver until I was nine. I have many memories of that house. As a little girl, I thought it was a huge house. It had lots of room for my sister and me to play. The basement of the house was turned into a huge play area for us. The two of us would spend hours downstairs playing games together. Often we would turn the basement into a classroom and play school. There were also times that the basement was transformed into a theater where we put on plays and concerts. Outside, in the backyard, we had a swing set and playhouse. In addition, three cats and a dog kept us entertained and busy. My sister and I always found a way to keep ourselves occupied.

Once my sister and I were old enough to attend school, we both went to Saint Vincent DePaul Catholic School in Denver. My mom eventually switched jobs and became the Director of Religious Education at our church—Church of the Risen Christ. The church was conveniently located just minutes from our house. When my mom changed jobs, my sister and I quickly adjusted to spending time at church with her. Even though we attended catholic school, we both enjoyed going to catechism classes and just being at the church. The church became like a second home to my sister and me. Through school and church, we made many friends and participated in numerous activities. Growing up in Denver, I never thought that one day I would trade the city for mountain living. I watched friends of mine move away, but under no circumstances thought that I would experience it myself. It was hard to imagine moving away from the house and community I had grown to know very well.

I'll never forget the day my parents told us that we were moving out of the city and to the mountains. I was in third grade. My father no longer had to legally live in Denver for his job, so they decided a move to the mountains was best for the family. After only knowing what it was like to live in a city, this news was definitely shocking. At the age of nine, I didn't know what to think. Of course, I was worried about the friends I had made. The thought of leaving them made me very sad. I was also nervous about having to start a new school. Not only would I be starting a new school, but I would be changing from a private school to a public school. To me, moving meant that I was going to have to start everything over again, and it was a little unsettling. I felt a mix of emotions leading up to the move.

In August 1999, I remember sitting out on the front lawn and watching the moving trucks pull up to our house in Denver. I sat and watched as box after box was carried onto the moving trucks. As I was sitting there watching, I think I was in denial of what was happening. It was hard for me to grasp that we were actually moving. When everything was loaded on the trucks, there was nothing left for us to do, and it was time to say goodbye to that Denver house. My sister and I piled into my mom's van with all our family pets. We then drove away from that house for the last time and began the journey towards Conifer, Colorado. A new chapter in our life was about to unfold. At that particular moment, I didn't realize it but moving to Conifer on that day was the best thing my parents ever did for us.

Looking back, moving to Conifer had so many positive influences on my life. Shortly after moving to Conifer, I started fourth grade at Marshdale Elementary. I then attended school in the community until I graduated from Conifer High School in 2008. From fourth grade all the way to my senior year of high school, I absolutely loved attending school in the community of Conifer. At school and within the community, I quickly met many friends. These people are still very important to me and part of my life now. Life was definitely different in the mountains, but I embraced it. My sister and I quickly got involved with extracurricular activities. As a family, we built an amazing life in the mountains, and we became attached to the community.

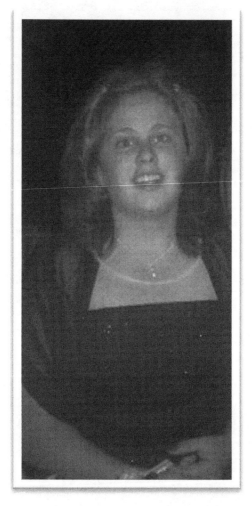

(Me at my Junior Prom in April 2007)

CHAPTER 2

The Appointment
that Changed Everything

While the information that is about to be revealed in the coming pages has technically affected me since birth, a major turning point in my life occurred when I was in high school. Oddly enough, this turning point happened when I decided I wanted to play lacrosse. Anyone who knows me knows that I am a major fan of the professional lacrosse team of Colorado—the Colorado Mammoth. The Colorado Mammoth were established when I was in eighth grade (2003). My dad took my sister, my friend, Aimee, and me to our first

Mammoth game. I was immediately hooked from that first game. I quickly realized that there is nothing like being at the Pepsi Center when the Mammoth are playing. The vibrant energy inside the stadium during a Mammoth game is contagious. In addition, the sport of lacrosse is fast and thrilling to watch. Also, the teenage girl in me didn't find it hard to watch some of the players. I left that first game a lacrosse fan and wanting to play the sport.

When I was sixteen and a junior at Conifer High School, I decided to try playing lacrosse. Before high school, I played soccer for a couple of years and even tried playing softball. After playing softball, I didn't play any other sports. One day, I realized that I wanted to experience what playing a sport in high school was like. Since I had become a lacrosse fan, I decided that would be the sport to try. At the time, Conifer High School did not have a girl's lacrosse team. Evergreen High School (which was not too far away) had a team, and some classmates of mine played on Evergreen's team. I had my mom attend an informational meeting with me, so that we could get all the paperwork that was needed to join the team. It made me excited to try something new. I was finally going to know what it was like to play lacrosse and be on a high school team.

As every athlete knows, one requirement for playing sports is a sports physical. Going to the doctor is something I have never enjoyed. In fact, visits to the doctor normally bring on some intense anxiety in me. Upon hearing that I would need a sports physical, I instantly had that feeling of anxiety. I don't know exactly what I was anxious about, but I could feel it. I think what always makes me anxious about visiting a doctor is my fear of being told bad news and my terrible phobia of needles. Despite my anxiety, I had my mom make me an appointment for a physical. My friends all assured me the appointment would be quick and easy. After a while, I actually believed that it was not going to be a big deal. It was just a sports physical after all. Little did I know that going in for a sports physical would change my life and stir up more emotions than I ever thought possible.

Before I knew it, my dad was driving me down to my appointment after school one day. My family had just changed insurance companies, so this was the first time that I would be visiting this doctor. I was a little nervous as we drove down the mountain, but I kept telling myself everything would be fine. We pulled into the parking lot, and my stomach dropped. I again told myself it would be fine and slowly got out of the car. I gathered my paperwork and walked into the building.

My dad and I found a place in the waiting room after I checked in. I sat and looked at a magazine as I waited. After a while, I heard my name called. I told my dad I would see him after the appointment and walked toward the nurse. My heart started to race as I walked toward her. I could feel my anxiety sinking in. The nurse checked all my vitals and then escorted me to the room to wait for the doctor. I waited and listened for the knock on the door signaling that the doctor was ready.

The knock on the door occurred and I muttered, "Come in." Suddenly, the doctor appeared, and the appointment began. Since it was my first time meeting with this particular doctor, she asked me several questions regarding my health history. I had answered about four questions and could tell something wasn't right after the fifth question. With a puzzled look on her face, she stopped asking questions and started the physical examination. After completing the examination, she asked if I had a parent waiting for me. I told her I had my father with me, and she requested that I go get him.

At that moment, I absolutely knew that something wasn't right. I told her I would go get my father, but what I desperately wanted to do was leave. To say that I didn't consider just walking out and telling my father that the appointment was over would be a lie. I walked as slow as I could out to the waiting room and told my dad that the doctor wanted to talk with him. He walked back with me to the examination room where the doctor was waiting. The doctor shut the door and thanked my father for coming to talk with her. She immediately told my father that she was concerned after conducting the physical examination. My father looked at me and asked me to leave the room. I looked at him and then at the doctor but couldn't say a word. Knowing that the doctor was concerned took my anxiety to a completely new level. I didn't want to leave the room at all. I wanted to stay in the room and listen to the conversation. My dad and the doctor looked at me in silence.

When I was finally able to break the silence, the first word I muttered was "No." My dad then pointed to the door and asked me to leave again. I knew that there was no point in arguing, so I walked toward the door and opened it. I walked out of the room and immediately put my ear up to the door to listen. There were people outside the door watching me, but at that moment, I didn't care. I was determined to know what was going on in the examination room. After putting my ear to the door, the next four words that I heard changed my life forever. I heard my dad say, "She has Turner syndrome." Those four words were all I had to hear. I don't know if I could ever fully describe how it felt to hear those words. It almost felt as if someone had punched me in the stomach, and I couldn't breathe. I stepped back and leaned against the wall on the opposite side of the door. I could not believe what I had just heard.

Minutes later, the door opened, and my father called me back into the room. The doctor explained that she wanted me to get a blood test done. She said that she was concerned and wanted to conduct a more detailed examination. I looked at her and asked if she intended to conduct the blood test that day. She nodded and said yes. At that moment, I couldn't hold it in any longer. I started crying and told her that I was absolutely terrified of needles and couldn't handle a blood test right away. After seeing my reaction, she tried to assure me everything was going to be fine. She gave me the option to come back for the blood test another time. Knowing that I didn't have to get the blood test done right away provided some relief. I thanked her and asked if it was okay to leave. She shook my hand, gave me my paperwork for lacrosse, and told me I could go home. Lacrosse was the last thing on my mind at that time, but I took the paperwork from her. My dad and I walked out of the examination room, and I immediately reached for my cell phone to call my mom.

When my mom answered my phone call, tears started to stream down my face even more. She asked me what was wrong, and all I could mutter was that the appointment didn't go as well as I had hoped. I also explained that I needed a blood test done. My mom knows how bad my phobia of needles is. I've always been extremely afraid of anything at the doctor's office that requires needles. After hearing that I needed a blood test, my mom tried to calm me down and tell me that everything was going to be ok. I wasn't able to muster up the courage to tell her what I had overheard my dad tell the doctor. I had no idea how I was going to broach that subject.

Once I got off the phone, my dad and I got into the car and left. I spent the entire car ride home thinking about what I was going to do next. What I heard my father tell the doctor made me feel a mix of emotions. I immediately had all sorts of questions. Besides wanting to know exactly what Turner syndrome was, I wanted to know if this was something I was born with. I also wanted to know who else knew that I had it, how it would affect (if at all) the rest of my life, and so many other things. Numerous thoughts and questions flooded my brain. The worst part was that I needed to figure out how I was going to get all this information. From what I could tell, my father didn't know I had overheard his conversation with the doctor. I knew I was going to need support from my parents. I just didn't know how I was going to tell them what I had heard. That part puzzled me throughout the car ride home.

When I got home, I ran to my bedroom, locked the door, and got my textbook out from genetics class. Coincidentally, I was taking a genetics class at school. I didn't have a computer in my bedroom, and there was only one in the house for the whole family. At that moment, I knew looking at my genetics textbook was the best way for me to try to get some information. I thought I remembered my teacher briefly talking about Turner syndrome on the day we discussed some genetic disorders. With shaking hands, I opened the book and went to the index to look up Turner syndrome. I then quickly flipped to the page listed in the index and immediately saw the information I was looking for. Even though I was nervous about what I was going to find out, I started reading my textbook.

I read all the information my textbook had about Turner syndrome. I was right in my thinking that it was a genetic disorder. The short and simple definition of Turner syndrome is that it is a genetic disorder in which a woman is born without one X chromosome or an X chromosome that is partially missing. Women have two X chromosomes while men have an X and a Y chromosome. I went on to read about physical characteristics that can be seen in women with Turner syndrome and other symptoms. I soaked in every piece of information that the textbook could give me. As I read, I began to get more emotional. I realized that I did have some of the physical characteristics and symptoms listed in the book.

After reading all the information I could, I put the textbook down. I sat on my bed, closed my eyes, and just took everything in. I could honestly not believe the events that had taken place in the past hours. At that moment, I desperately wanted to open my eyes and realize that everything was just a dream. I opened my eyes and stared at the ceiling. I thought about what I was going to do next. One thing I knew is that I wanted to talk with my mother about this situation. My mother would definitely have some of the answers I was searching for. I just didn't know how I was going to tell her that I knew I had Turner syndrome.

The moment to talk with my mother came the next morning. When I have something I need to talk about, I can't hold it in very long. I'm the kind of person that likes to talk about things quickly. I remember waking up the morning after the doctor's appointment and deciding that I wanted to talk with mom before leaving for school. My sister and I were blessed to have a mother who cooked us breakfast every morning before school. That day, my mom was cooking breakfast, and I was sitting at the kitchen table getting ready for school. She brought up the doctor's appointment. At that moment, I just blurted out, "Do I have Turner syndrome?" My mom paused, looked at me, and quickly said, "Yes, you do have a form of it. That is why the doctor wants to do some blood tests." I can't remember the rest of our conversation word for word. It took time for me to process the answer my mother gave me. I know that we discussed I had a form of Turner syndrome, and that my parents had known about it since my birth. According to my mother, doctors had told her I had Mosaic Turner syndrome. To this day, I can't remember how I explained to my mom why I was asking about Turner syndrome. I know that I didn't tell her about the conversation I had overheard at the doctor's. Overall, I was glad that I went to school that morning with some answers. I finally felt like I had some of the answers I longed for.

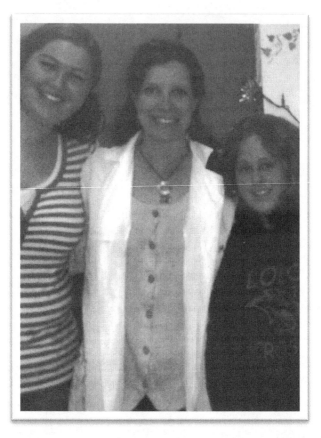

(My good friend, Rachelle, and me with Mrs. Stricker at Conifer High School. We both were fortunate to have Mrs. Stricker as a teacher for many Science classes throughout our time at Conifer)

CHAPTER 3

The Journey
I Never Expected

After getting some of the answers I wanted, the next thing going through my mind was how and if I was going to tell my friends about my diagnosis. I knew I didn't need to tell them, and that no one was forcing me to. However, I felt that it was going to be hard to keep the information a secret forever. Just like I knew I would need my parents' support, I knew I would also need some support from friends. The fact that I have Turner syndrome was not something I planned to tell everyone right away, but I decided there were a couple of friends I wanted to tell. I just didn't know the best way to tell those friends.

My friend Aimee was the first friend I told about the doctor's appointment. Aimee knew I had anxiety about going to the doctor's, so she asked how it went the next morning. Her question made it easy for me to tell her everything. I explained that I had found out I had Turner syndrome and about the information I had read in my textbook. I also told her about the conversation I had with my mother that morning. I remember being extremely nervous when I was talking to Aimee. The nerves were nothing against her. She had been my friend since elementary school, and we were extremely close. We told each other everything. I was mostly nervous about the fact that she was the first person I was telling this information to. At that particular moment, I was revealing some extremely personal information. I guess I was nervous about the reaction I was going to get. When all was said and done, Aimee reacted to the information I shared in the way I thought she would. She asked me how I was doing and told me everything was going to be ok. In the end, I was very thankful to Aimee and happy to have her as part of my support system.

Aimee was the only friend I told about that doctor's appointment (and what I found out) for a while. I felt like I needed time to process and think about everything. Finding out I had Turner syndrome was literally like embarking on a journey I never expected. Initially, the hardest part about the journey was that each day something reminded me that I have Turner syndrome. I could not go a day without being reminded somehow about my condition. Whether it was genetics class, a TV show with a doctor, or even random conversations, something would trigger my memory about it every day. Even though I knew the reminders were not intentional or anyone's fault, they were difficult to deal with at first. I didn't like thinking about the fact that I have Turner syndrome each day. Thinking about it triggered a wide range of emotions. After my conversation with Aimee, I determined that I needed some time to begin navigating through my new journey before I opened up to other people. At that particular time, I was still learning what

Turner syndrome was. I also was trying to work through the anxiety I had about upcoming visits to the doctor.

Within a couple days after my sports physical, I decided that I was not going to play lacrosse that season. For many reasons, I just couldn't get myself to officially join the team. I felt like the most important thing for me, at that time, was to process the information I had just learned. To be honest, I think I was also nervous about what would happen with my blood work. I worried about the results that would come from it. Even though I had been excited about playing a high school sport, I didn't think adding lacrosse to my schedule was a good idea at that time. Ultimately, I believed that I had other things to work through before I played a sport.

It took some time, but my mom was eventually able to get me back to the doctor's office to get the blood work done. I'll spare all the details about how that visit went. Any visit to the doctor's that involves needles is always one that makes me very anxious. Let's just say it was not a fun visit and definitely involved many tears.

After getting the blood test, my mother was referred to a specialist at a children's hospital for me. My primary care physician told my parents it would be important for me to see a specialist who knew more about Turner syndrome and could monitor me. I never expected to see a specialist.

When the blood work was done, my mom scheduled the appointment for me to go to the children's hospital. That appointment marked the first time I had been to the children's hospital in Denver. In addition, it was the first time I had seen a specialist of any kind. Walking into that appointment, I had no idea what to expect. I, of course, was extremely nervous, but I tried to find comfort in the fact that I had my mother accompanying me to the appointment. We sat in the waiting room and shortly after, we were called back into the examination room. My anxiety kicked in as soon as I heard my name called. I would have done anything to leave the hospital at that moment. The nurse walked us in to the room and then told us that the doctor would be with us shortly.

Before I knew it, there was a knock on the door. The doctor walked in and my first impression of her was good. She shook my hand and was pleasant. We then got talking about why I was there and the recent blood tests I had done. We were there for about an hour or so. I don't know what I was exactly expecting to hear from this specialist, but I most definitely was not expecting to hear I had more medical testing ahead of me. The specialist explained that with my age and my condition, it was important to do some tests to ensure I didn't have any of the health complications associated with Turner syndrome and that everything in my body was functioning normally. I left that doctor's appointment knowing I needed more blood tests, X-rays, ultrasounds, a heart test, and more. To say that I was overwhelmed leaving that doctor's appointment was an understatement. For someone who gets anxious about doctor's appointments, I wasn't too happy about the tests I needed to get done.

The medical tests were done either at my primary care physician's office or at the children's hospital. It took three appointments to get all the tests done. Once the tests were done, I had to go back to the specialist to discuss the results. The day my mom and I went back to meet with the specialist again, my emotions got the best of me. For one thing, I didn't like missing school. I was taking Advanced Placement (AP) classes, and those classes were always difficult to miss. I took my classes very seriously. The day of the appointment, I was already frustrated because I knew I'd be leaving during my AP History class. I grew even more frustrated the minute my history teacher's phone rang, and I was told to go to the office. Even though I didn't want to, I walked down to the office, met my mom, and went out to the car with her. I got in the car, and the way I acted clearly showed my mom I was mad. I threw my backpack on the back seat and slammed the door very loudly. At that moment, my mom looked at me and said in a serious tone, "If you don't want to do this, I'll just let you go back to school." I muttered, "Let's go and get this over with" and then kept quiet. I'm not proud of how I acted that day. As I said, I let my emotions get the best of me. Walking out to the car that day triggered many different emotions within me.

Stress, anger, and anxiety were just some of the emotions I started fluctuating between.

As we drove down to the appointment, I tried to get my emotions under control. I knew I shouldn't be taking my frustration out on others. I also knew that I was thankful and happy to have my mom by my side. By the time we pulled into the hospital's parking lot, I was calmer, but I still didn't want to get out of the car. Going into the doctor's appointment was the last thing I wanted to do. I thought about the previous appointment I had at the hospital, and how I walked out knowing more medical tests needed to be done. I prayed for good news as I walked into the building. It was my hope that this appointment would end on a better note than my last one.

As usual, my mom and I were escorted back to the examination room by a nurse after she took my weight and height. The doctor quickly came in, and we immediately began talking about the tests that were completed. Some of the first words the specialist said were, "I am going to just say this to have it out there. I know you know this already, but you definitely have a form of Turner syndrome." My mom and I both looked at each other, and I nodded my head. I looked at the doctor and said, "All right, what does all this mean?" The doctor began to explain how overall my test results did not show any major red flags. I was then told that I would never have a normal menstrual cycle. It was explained that not having a normal menstrual cycle would obviously mean that naturally conceiving a child would be difficult for me. The specialist said if I wanted to have children someday, other conversations would need to happen in order to go over my options.

Learning that having children in the future would be difficult for me was indescribable. My mother immediately started to cry. I was completely speechless. I later found out that my mother already knew pregnancy would be hard for me. However, I think hearing it again and having me hear it was what made it difficult for her. I could not think of anything to say at that moment. The doctor acknowledged that this was difficult and that eventually other conversations about my options may be helpful. There was not much else to say on that topic after that. I didn't even know what to say, and I personally wanted the conversation to move on as quickly as possible. I knew I was not ready to have those discussions about pregnancy yet. Before having any of those conversations, I first wanted to process the information I had just learned.

The conversation then shifted to, of all things, my height. The doctor explained that my short stature was a symptom of Turner syndrome. I was told that growth hormones were an option for me, if I wanted, but this decision would have to be made pretty quickly because of my age. By this time, we had been talking for almost an hour, and my brain was on overload. I didn't even know what to think. To be honest, I didn't even know growth hormones existed before the appointment, and now I had to decide if I wanted them. I then also had to think about when conversations regarding my options with pregnancy should happen. My mind was once again flooded with numerous thoughts that I couldn't sort out. I was pretty sure at that moment that I did not want growth hormones. I told the doctor that I would think about it and let them know if I wanted to take them.

On the way home from the hospital, I talked with my mother to try to get some more of my looming questions answered. One of the things I asked her was if I had been told I had Turner syndrome before. I found out that she had a talk with me when I was younger, but that she didn't use the term Turner syndrome. My mother said that at one point it was explained to me that having a child on my own might not be possible, and that I would eventually need to see a doctor about it. After my mother told me this, I could vaguely remember that conversation. I then asked my mother how I reacted to that news. She told me I just responded by saying I would then adopt children. According to my mother, hearing that news when I was younger didn't really bother me. Looking back, I wonder if the fact that I didn't have a negative reaction to that conversation is why I don't remember much of it. I know the conversation happened but couldn't tell you word for word what was said. In the end, being able to remember some of it and knowing that my mother did talk with me gave me a sense of relief. My mom and I talked the entire ride home, and I felt like I got some more answers.

Later that day, I had an epiphany while I was in my bedroom by myself. I sat on my bed and tried to process all the information the doctor had just told me. As I was thinking about everything, I got a little emotional. A steady stream of tears started to fall down my face. All of a sudden, I realized I had a choice to make. I could let myself get really emotional, and let my sadness consume me; or I could decide to accept my diagnosis and not let it define me. In the end, I realized that there was nothing I could do to change what the doctor said. Nothing could be done to change the fact that I have Turner syndrome. Nothing could be done to change the symptoms of Turner syndrome that I have. It was then that I decided I was going to accept everything and move on. I determined there was no point in getting emotional over everything and letting it consume me. Focusing my energy on accepting everything seemed like the better option. After all, Turner syndrome would not change the fact that I was still the same old Kelsey.

I didn't know it in the moment, but on that day, I "reframed" the situation I was in. Reframing by definition means, "Taking a negative comment or situation and changing your perspective on it so that you can move on (Flippen Group, 2015, p. 46)."As I sat in my bedroom that day, I decided I wanted to move on and not let my diagnosis change me. It may not seem like it but "reframing" the situation and determining that Turner syndrome wasn't going to define me was one of the most difficult things I ever had to do. It is so much easier said than done. I knew that if I dwelled on everything and let my emotions consume me, it would turn me into a different person. I was determined not to let anything have a negative impact on me.

Deciding that I was not going to let this news change me obviously helped me develop a positive mindset and move on easier. About a week or so after my last visit to the children's hospital, I remember a friend asking me a question I wondered if I would hear. It happened one morning during our STAR time. STAR time occurred a couple of times a week before school. It was a time when students could go visit with any teachers to discuss assignments or get additional help. Students could also go to the library to work on assignments during that time. On this particular morning, my friend and I were in the classroom of our science teacher, Mrs. Stricker, who taught genetics. I remember we were working on an assignment and while we were working, my friend asked me if I was ok. She then went on to explain that she had noticed I had been going to the doctor's a lot recently and just wanted to know if I was ok. While I appreciated my friend's concern, I was rather caught off guard by it. At that moment, I had no idea what I was going to say. I stopped working on the assignment, took a deep breath, and told her about my condition. She was the second friend I told that I had Turner syndrome. She, like my friend Aimee, reacted in a very positive way. I knew that if I had not "reframed" the situation and had a more positive mindset, that moment would not have gone as well as it did.

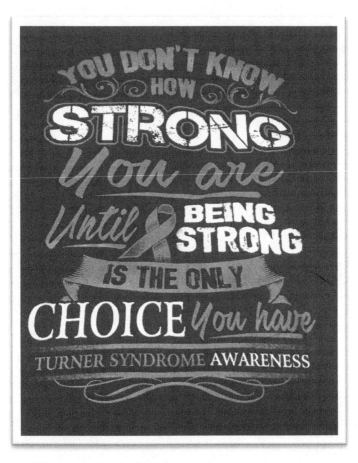

(Photograph of a Turner syndrome awareness t-shirt I purchased)

CHAPTER 4

What Did It All Mean?

Finding out that I had Turner syndrome provided me with an answer to a question I had thought about my entire life (until I learned about the diagnosis). Throughout my life, I have been asked numerous times why I was short. People who have met my entire immediate family know that I am by far the shortest. My father is 6'5", my mom is 5'8", and my sister is 5'10". It didn't make sense to some people how I was so much shorter than them. Honestly, I didn't blame people for asking that question because I knew it didn't make sense. I wondered about it pretty often myself.

Growing up, there was a period when I was taller than my younger sister was. There was also a period when we were the same height. Both of those phases were very short lived. I think by the time I went to middle school, my sister was taller than me. I was always told that I had inherited the short gene from my mom's side of the family. My maternal grandmother was very short as well. After being given that explanation, I lived with it. When people asked me why I was so short, I just smiled and told them my grandmother was very short. I didn't think twice about giving that answer.

After learning about my diagnosis, I realized I finally had an answer to that question, which was so frequently asked of me. Turner syndrome most definitely plays a part in why I am short. I chose not to take the growth hormones, and today, I am five feet tall. I spent a lot of time contemplating if I was going to take the hormones. In the end, I decided that God made me the way I was, and I didn't want to change it. Being short never really mattered to me or bothered me at all. In fact, I grew to like it. I quickly learned that being short actually had benefits. To this day, I do not regret the decision I made not to take the growth hormones. I am thankful that the decision regarding the hormones was left to me. At five feet, I may be the shortest in my immediate family, but it was good to finally have a better understanding of why I was short.

Now that I know Turner syndrome plays a part in my short stature, it makes it a little different when someone asks me why I am so short compared to the rest of my family. When I am asked that question now, it immediately makes me think about the fact that I have Turner syndrome. Even though I know the real answer to that question, I never felt comfortable with giving the answer until I was twenty-eight. While I was not ashamed of the real answer to the question, I guess I just didn't want to reveal that I had Turner syndrome to someone that way. I didn't want to just come out and say, "Well, I'm short because I have Turner syndrome." After I learned about my diagnosis, if I told anyone that I have Turner syndrome, it was important to me to spend time explaining some things to them. I liked to give some background information about what it is, and a little about how I found out about having it. I felt better talking to someone about having Turner syndrome when I initiated the conversation and could tell them things on my terms. Wanting to tell people things on my own terms is why I usually stuck with my generic, "I inherited the short gene from my mom's side of the family," answer to that question. If I was asked that question today, I would without a doubt be comfortable going into more detail about the real answer to that question. I no longer hold back any information.

Finding out about my diagnosis not only provided me with some clarification on my short stature, it also, initially, made a specific question difficult for me to hear. That question was if I wanted to have kids. I think there are many women who can relate to being asked that question at some point in their lives by family or friends. I, of course, was asked this question prior to learning about my diagnosis but have been asked it since then as well. My answer to this question hasn't changed since I learned I have Turner syndrome. I have always wanted to be a mother. The hard part of being asked if I wanted kids someday is that when it's brought up, I immediately think about the fact that a natural pregnancy may not be an option for me. Initially it was very difficult to be reminded of that, but I tried not to let myself get wrapped up in the emotions. If I am asked the question about kids, I always answer yes because it is true. Nothing will change the fact that I would love to be a mother. I believe when the time is right, I will be blessed with a child or children somehow. As time went on, having that specific question brought up became easier. Yes, it is still sometimes difficult to think about how Turner syndrome can affect pregnancies, but now I am at a better place with everything. Today, being asked if I want kids does not trigger as many emotions.

Whether it was providing me with an answer to a question or making a question difficult to hear, finding out about my diagnosis made me reflect a lot and want to learn more. I turned to the Internet to help me gain more knowledge about my condition. Throughout the years, I have done numerous Internet searches on Turner syndrome and Mosaic Turner syndrome. I'll never forget the day I came across a post on a forum after searching Mosaic Turner syndrome. The post was by a woman who had just found out her unborn child had Mosaic Turner syndrome. She had just been to the doctor and received the news through amniocentesis. On her post, she stated that she was scared and didn't know what to do. She requested advice on whether or not to continue with her pregnancy. I immediately started reading the responses she received. Thankfully, there were women who responded to her saying that Mosaic Turner syndrome really wasn't a big deal, and that her daughter would live a normal life.

After reading that post on the Internet, I thought about it a lot. My mom also found out I had Mosaic Turner syndrome through amniocentesis while she was pregnant. I couldn't help but think about my mom, and how she felt when she learned about my diagnosis. I also thought about the life I had lived up until that point. When I read this post, I was in my late twenties. The post was four–years-old, but if it had been recent, I would have responded (like the other women who did) and explained that Mosaic Turner syndrome really is not a big deal. Having it did not stop me from living the life I wanted to. I felt blessed and thankful to be living the life I was. Doing research showed me such a wide range of reading material on Turner syndrome, and I continued to read as much as I could.

Numerous articles I found online describe the different forms of Turner syndrome. There are different forms of Turner syndrome that a woman can have. One form of Turner syndrome occurs when a woman is completely missing an X chromosome. Women who are completely missing an X chromosome have what is called "classic Turner syndrome." Another form of Turner syndrome is when the X chromosome is absent in some cells but not all of them. Mosaic Turner syndrome is the term used to describe the form in which the X chromosome is not absent in all cells. Having Mosaic Turner syndrome can result in milder symptoms than other forms of the disorder. Turner syndrome affects one in every 2500 girls born. It is named after Dr. Henry Turner who discovered it in

1938. Dr. Turner was one of the first doctors to report on the disorder in literature.

Overall, what I have gathered from doing my own research on Turner syndrome is that it can affect girls and women differently. Some women may have more symptoms than other women. Symptoms can include wide or web-like neck, low-set ears, low hairline at the back of the neck, and arms that turn outward at the elbow. Turner syndrome can also cause some health complications. Complications can include heart problems, high blood pressure, hearing loss, kidney problems, autoimmune disorders, vision problems, and skeletal problems. As mentioned previously, each case of Turner syndrome is unique. There are lots of articles and websites with information about Turner syndrome. However, I found that there were not a lot of published books about it. Most of the information I have gained about Turner syndrome has been from reading articles and journals online.

While doing an Internet search on Turner syndrome, most sources will say that women affected by it will have normal intelligence, but there is a chance of learning difficulties, behavior problems, and even social problems. After reading those things for the first time, I spent time reflecting and thinking about what being a student was like for me. I was in high school when I first read that women with Turner syndrome can have learning difficulties. It made me a little nervous about starting college, but, in the end, I knew I was a good student. At no point during my educational career did it show that I had learning difficulties. As far as social and behavior problems go, I felt those were things I did not have either (although my mom may not 100 percent agree on the behavior part 😅).

Doing research on my condition sometimes triggered difficult emotions. At times, it was hard to read information about Turner syndrome. Even though it was difficult, I was motivated to do research to help me gain a better understanding of everything. To me, it was important to learn as much as I could about my condition. Spending time doing some research allowed me to understand what having Turner syndrome really meant.

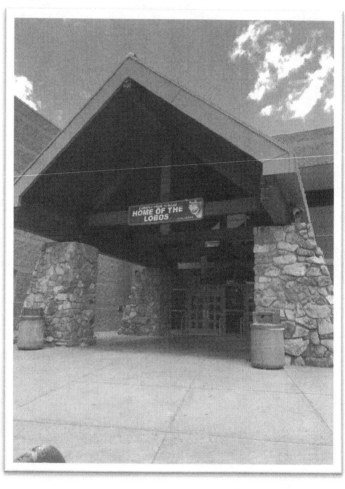

(Front entrance to Conifer High School)

CHAPTER 5

Navigating Through High School

One of the best things that happened to me during my time at Conifer High School was being selected as a peer coach for the Unified Physical Education (P.E.) program. This program paired me with an individual with disabilities who also attended Conifer, and together we worked to prepare for Special Olympics events. At least three times a week, I would attend gym class with this student where we would work together to prepare for the events. We did everything from bowling to track and field. One of the individuals I coached in the

Unified P.E. program is named Kathleen. By working together in PE, Kathleen quickly became a close friend, and I will forever cherish the time I was her coach.

Kathleen helped me through some difficult times in high school. As I've said previously, I struggled emotionally after I learned I had Turner syndrome. If I was having a rough day, Kathleen would quickly notice it. She would always ask me, "Are you ok buddy?" If I told her I was ok but just having a rough day, often her response was, "Buddy, everything will be ok. Smile!" After being told those words, I couldn't help but smile. Through the years that I worked with Kathleen, she taught me so much. I helped prepare her for Special Olympics events but she helped me in ways she will never know. To this day, Kathleen is still a very important part of my life.

August 2007 was the start of my senior year at Conifer High School. I was once again a part of the Unified P.E. program at Conifer. I was going on my second year as producer of the school news show "Lobotrax" and was co-president of the Key Club. I started my senior year happy with my life at Conifer High School. I loved all the programs I was involved with, and overall I liked school. I was probably one of the only high school seniors in America who could say that I did not start senior year with "senioritis." I started that school year excited to see what it would bring. I knew I had some big decisions ahead of me such as what college I would attend, and what I would major in. As the school year started, my goal was to just embrace senior year and not rush anything. I was not in a hurry to graduate and leave high school behind. I wanted to make senior year as amazing as I could.

I loved being a part of the Unified P.E. program and couldn't imagine doing anything else. Prior to my senior year, I entertained the idea of going to college for science (since I was interested in genetics and forensic science) or even business. However, senior year was when it really occurred to me as to which path I needed to take in college. It became clear to me that helping individuals with disabilities was my passion. I immediately started research on colleges and the programs they had to offer.

In October 2007, my mom took me and some of my friends to visit the University of Northern Colorado (UNC). From the moment I set foot on the campus, I was immediately hooked. Everything about the campus appealed to me. Every person I interacted with on campus that day was very nice and expressed how much they enjoyed going to UNC. The buildings on campus and the surrounding areas was beautiful. I could see myself living in the dorm rooms I saw. The campus wasn't too big, and I learned the class sizes were pretty small. Everything I saw at UNC that day was what I had hoped for in a college. The list of positive things I saw about UNC in just one visit went on and on.

At an informational meeting, I learned that my ACT scores paired with my overall GPA from high school guaranteed me admission into UNC. Once I learned that, my decision was set. I left UNC that October day knowing I would be back in ten months to start my undergraduate degree.

I knew I was going to attend UNC to major in special education. It just seemed like it was the right thing for me to do. To be honest, I didn't even consider any other colleges. The more I thought about it and reflected on going to UNC, I grew excited about my decision.

During my senior year, I decided to try playing lacrosse again. That year, Conifer was forming the first ever girls' varsity and junior varsity lacrosse teams. My sister and I both ended up trying out for the teams. That year, I played on the varsity team. I finally got to experience playing a high school sport, and I enjoyed every minute. My teammates became close friends quickly. It was an awesome experience to play a sport I enjoy with my friends. I think one of my favorite memories from that year was winning the game against our rival high school. I'll always be thankful that I took the opportunity to be a part of Conifer High School's first ever girls varsity lacrosse team.

I will never forget the day that really solidified my decision to go into special education. Some teachers can tell you a defining moment in their lives when they knew they wanted to go into education. That moment for me happened near the end of my senior year at Conifer. My Unified P.E. class went to compete in a track and field meet. That day brought many emotions. It was the last event I would be coaching Kathleen at. I could not believe that my time in the Unified P.E. program (and at Conifer High School) was ending. It made me sad to think about not being Kathleen's coach anymore. I was determined to make the most of the day though.

The day involved me helping Kathleen compete in various track and field events. We had been practicing the different events in P.E. class for many weeks. Throughout the time that we were preparing for the meet, I always did the running with Kathleen. She didn't like to practice running events unless I was doing it with her. No matter what I tried in class, Kathleen would not run by herself. When it was time for the fifty-yard dash at the meet, I didn't know what to expect. I walked her over to the starting line and spoke with someone running the event. One of the individuals in charge gave me permission to run beside Kathleen, if needed. Before the event started, I pulled her aside and asked if she was comfortable running by herself, or if she wanted me to run with her. She looked at me and said something along the lines of, "Buddy, I know I can do it by myself now." I gave her a hug, and I told her I would go wait for her at the finish line. Quickly, I found a good spot where I could watch the race. The whistle blew, and Kathleen started running pretty fast. I started clapping and cheering loudly for her. Kathleen ran all the way to the finish line but didn't stop there. She went right past it and came to give me a huge hug. At that particular moment, it became clear to me that I was making the right decision to major in special education. I knew without a doubt that it was the right career path for me.

Looking back at my journey through high school, I believe everything happened the way it did for a reason. I think there is a reason I found out about having Turner syndrome when I was taking genetics class. Surprisingly enough, the semester I took genetics class was the first semester it was ever offered at Conifer. The teacher, who taught the class, Mrs. Stricker, had been my science teacher for a semester of earth science and a year of biology previously. I decided to take genetics because it was a topic that interested me, and I thought Mrs. Stricker was an amazing teacher. I could not be happier that I chose to take that class. Being in that class when I found out about my diagnosis helped me in many ways. The content that I learned in that class helped me gain a better understanding of everything the doctors were telling me. In addition, Mrs. Stricker also found out I had Turner syndrome. I don't remember exactly how I told her, but I think it was on the same day I told my friend everything in her classroom. She was an adult I trusted, so I was fine that she knew. It actually made me feel a little better to have her know I had Turner syndrome. I cannot imagine what it would have been like if I hadn't taken genetics class in my junior year.

I also think there was a reason I was accepted into the Unified P.E. program at Conifer. In order to be part of the program, I had to be interviewed by the physical education teacher because there were a limited number of spots. Being a part of the Unified P.E. program not only helped me decide the career path I wanted to follow, it also helped me get through some tough times in high school. Being a coach and mentor to other students was such a rewarding experience. In fact, I found it so rewarding that I spent any free time I had helping the students I coached in their academic classes as well. I quickly got to know the special education staff at Conifer High School and loved helping them in any way I could. I'm very thankful I was given the opportunity to be a part of the Unified P.E. program.

As I sat at my high school graduation ceremony on May 24, 2008, I couldn't believe I was at that point in my life. It was hard to comprehend that four years at Conifer High School had already passed. After the graduation ceremony, I spent the day at numerous parties with friends. Throughout the day as I spent time with friends, it hit me that our time as students at Conifer High School was over. It was hard for me to think about not going back to high school in August. I had so many emotions as I thought about starting college in the fall. I was excited to see what college was about, but I was also nervous about leaving my friends and starting a new journey. In less than two months, I would be a University of Northern Colorado Bear. It was hard for me to grasp the fact that I was about to be a college student.

There is no denying that navigating through my last two years of high school had some challenges. I never expected to find out that I have a genetic disorder at the age of sixteen. As I have said though, I do think everything happened the way that it did for a reason. As odd as it may seem, being in the genetics class and Unified P.E. program when I found out about my diagnosis really helped me. I do believe that despite the challenges I faced, I made the most out of my last two years at high school. Overall, my experience as a Conifer High School student was a good one. Throughout the four years I was a student at Conifer, I was proud to call myself a Conifer High School Lobo.

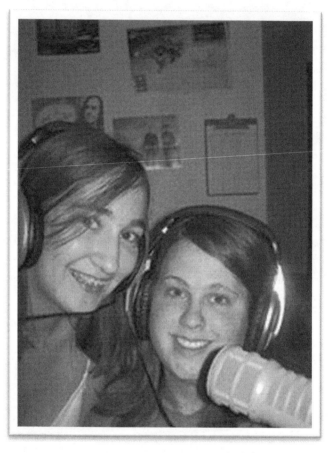

(Kelsey Poole and me in the UNC Student Radio studio-September 2010)

CHAPTER 6

From Conifer High School Lobo to University of Northern Colorado Bear

The start of my freshman year of college at the University of Northern Colorado was the beginning of an incredible four-year journey. While it was an incredible journey, I was extremely nervous to start it. I'll never forget the day I moved into my dorm as a freshmen at UNC. As I drove away from my parents' house that day and headed towards Greeley, I fought back tears and felt sick to my stomach. My car was packed with all my belongings, and my mom was in the passenger seat. My dad followed us in his car. Even though I knew I wasn't saying goodbye to Conifer forever, I was nervous. It made me nervous to think that I was officially a college student and would be living on my own. I loved living in Conifer and wasn't ready to leave it. Thankfully, UNC was less than a two-hour drive from Conifer.

After arriving in Greeley, both my parents helped me unload my car and get my dorm room organized. Looking at my dorm room, it was hard for me to believe that the small space in front of me was my new room. It helped that my roommate was a friend from high school. All day, I dreaded the time that my parents would leave. I think what I worried about the most was how emotional it would be. I knew that if my parents started crying, I would too. When it was time to say goodbye, of course it was emotional. In the end, it wasn't as bad as I thought it was going to be. After a week or so, I was pretty adjusted to college life and enjoying it. It didn't take long for me to realize that it was kind of fun to be living on my own.

Shortly into my freshman year, my roommate, Margaret (who I went to high school with), and I met Kelsey Poole. Kelsey very quickly became a close friend. She was also a freshman and majoring in elementary education. Margaret was majoring in early childhood education, so Kelsey Poole fit right in with us. Since all three of us were majoring in education, we took some of the same classes together. Kelsey Poole spent so much time in the dorm room Margaret and I shared that she eventually moved most of her belongings into our room. The three of us ended up cramming all our belongings into a room that some would say was small for two people, but we had fun with it. After all, you only live once, right? I still don't know how we weren't caught for having three people living in that room.

Kelsey, Margaret, and I remained roommates throughout our entire college careers. We lived in many dorm rooms and apartments together. Looking back, I am so happy I had them both with me throughout all four years of college.

Since the three of us were studying to become teachers, we were able to support each other through our education classes. We also shared many of the same interests, which made it fun. Living together was an adventure for sure.

A couple years into college, Kelsey and I became co-hosts of a radio show for UNC Student Radio. In the fall of 2010, we were approached by the General Manager of UNC Student Radio at an event on campus. He told us that we should consider hosting a radio show, and that got Kelsey and me thinking about it. Before we knew it, two DJs from the station had us as guests on their show. After that, Kelsey and I agreed to host a weekly show. By the end of September 2010, our radio show, K Fusion, was on the air.

Going into college, I never thought that I would become a co-host of a radio show. It was one of the best experiences of my college career. Kelsey and I loved every minute of hosting K Fusion. When I think about college, some of my favorite memories are the nights the two of us would blast the music in the studio and sing along to the songs. We, of course, would always make sure our microphones were on mute to avoid being heard on air. I think it's safe to say that we would have lost listeners if our singing voices had been heard on the air.

One of my favorite things about being involved with UNC Student Radio was how relaxing it was. Our radio show was always on Thursday nights. Hosting a weekly radio show helped motivate Kelsey and me through each week. As we walked into the studio each Thursday night, it was always refreshing to know that Friday was so close. We both found that hosting our radio show was a fun way to bring each school week to a close. It didn't matter what had happened throughout the week or even that day. When we walked into the studio, it was left at the door. For an hour, we were able to listen to some of our favorite music, interact with our listeners, and just have fun. Thursday nights in the studio were something we always looked forward to. I couldn't imagine having any other co-host.

Eventually, I did tell Kelsey Poole about me having Turner syndrome. I remember that I was less anxious about telling her than I was about telling other friends. By the time I told Kelsey Poole, I had known about my diagnosis for a while. It wasn't new information, and I felt more comfortable with everything. After I told Kelsey Poole, I was happy that I had opened up to her. She was the first friend from college that I told about my diagnosis. Just like Aimee, Kelsey reacted to the information in a positive way. From that point on, she was a great support for me when I needed it.

Overall, I would say that I had an amazing college experience at UNC. Throughout the four years that I was in college, I was reminded in numerous ways that I had made the right decision by coming to UNC. I wouldn't change a thing about my college experience. Over the years, I made amazing friends, enjoyed the classes I took, had wonderful professors, and had so many awesome opportunities. Without a doubt, every minute I had at UNC taught me a lot and really prepared me for a career in education. I could not be more proud to be a UNC Bear.

My time as a college student seemed to fly by and before I knew it, my journey at UNC ended. On May 5, 2012, I officially celebrated the end of my undergraduate college career and graduated from UNC. It was such an amazing feeling to stand on that stage and receive my diploma. As I stood on that stage, I thought about the past four years and what it meant to me. After four years of hard work that involved not only taking classes but also holding down jobs, I was finally getting my degree. I could not have been more excited to graduate from UNC. On that particular day, I did not know exactly what the future had in store for me. However, it didn't take long for me to figure out what my next adventure would be.

Prior to graduating from college, I had spent some time looking for jobs. I attended a teaching fair at UNC and filled out applications online. While looking for jobs, I tried to find positions as close to Conifer as I could. My overall goal was to get a job within the mountain community. I wanted to go back to the Conifer area because I loved the small mountain town feel. When I started looking for jobs though, I knew that I was possibly going to have to move further away if I was offered a job somewhere else. Even though I filled out applications online and attended the teaching fair, I did not have a job secured. It was a little unnerving not to have something secured before graduating but I prayed that the right job would come my way. The answer to my prayers came almost exactly a month after graduating from college.

After graduating from college, I was a paraprofessional for a month at the school I student taught at in Evergreen, Colorado. They hired me to work in the month of May as a paraprofessional. One morning before going to work, I was spending some time looking for jobs and came across an opening at Deer Creek Elementary school in Bailey, CO. Bailey is a town that is not far from Conifer. I was immediately excited because it was exactly what I was looking for—a job close to Conifer. I filled out an application before going to work. That day, while I was at work, I received a call asking me to come in for an interview. I left work that day with an interview set up, and I couldn't have been more excited. I couldn't wait to get home and tell my mom I had an interview.

Near the end of May 2012 was when I had my interview at Deer Creek Elementary in Bailey. Prior to interviewing at the school, I had never been in the building, but I had driven past it before. I was of course nervous while going to the interview but was also excited. This was the first interview I would have at one of the mountain schools close to Conifer. I was hoping for the best as I walked into the interview. I really wanted it to go well.

The principal, assistant principal, and one of the special education teachers in the building were the ones who interviewed me. Shortly after I started the interview, I knew Deer Creek was the school I wanted to be at. All three of the staff members who interviewed me made me feel welcome and showed me what a great place Deer Creek was. Once the four of us were done talking, the special education teacher who helped with the interview, Maurita, showed me around the school. Getting a chance to see the school and talk with Maurita made me want the job even more. From the short amount of time I interacted with her, I knew she would make an amazing teammate. I walked out of that interview praying that I would get the opportunity to be part of the staff at Deer Creek. Once I got back to my car, the first thing I did was call my mom and tell her how much I wanted the job. As I mentioned previously, I had been to a job fair before and interviewed at various Colorado school districts. I did not feel the same way after the interviews at the job fair as I did after my interview at Deer Creek. The interview at Deer Creek left me very excited. As I drove home, I felt I had done pretty well at the interview and hoped the staff members who interviewed me felt the same. Something about Deer Creek just felt right to me.

June 6, 2012, almost a month after graduation, was when I received my official job offer at Deer Creek. That summer, I worked at a summer camp for individuals with disabilities. Kathleen, my friend from high school who I coached in the Unified P.E. program, attended this camp. On the particular day that I received my job offer, I was working, and Kathleen was with me. Sometimes, I would spend some time with Kathleen after camp, so she would leave with me at the end of the day. On June 6, 2012, Kathleen and I were walking out to my car, and I realized I had a voicemail from a number I didn't recognize. Thinking that it could be someone from Deer Creek, I immediately listened to it. The voicemail was from Kay, the Assistant Principal at Deer Creek, offering me the job. After hearing that I had been offered the job, I immediately was overcome with excitement. I looked at Kathleen and screamed with excitement, "I am going to be a teacher!" It was hard for me to contain my happiness. Kathleen immediately shouted, "Way to go buddy." At that moment, I could not have been more excited or happy. A new chapter of my life was about to begin and I couldn't wait.

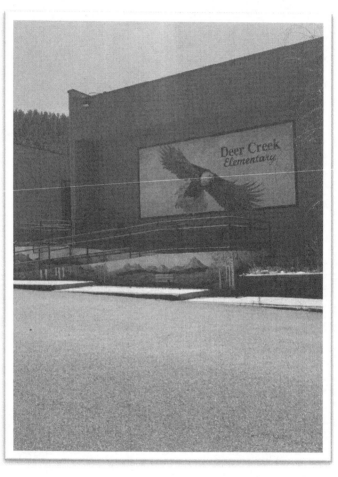

(Deer Creek Elementary School- Bailey, Colorado)

CHAPTER 7

Teacher Life

August 2012 marked the start of my teaching career. As I drove to school that first day, I remember feeling a mix of emotions. Of course, I was excited, but I also was a little nervous. I had done a lot of teaching throughout my four years of college, but this time I was going to have my own classroom. Before, I had a cooperating (or host) teacher who helped me with some of the responsibilities of the classroom and offered advice. Now, I was officially a teacher and had a classroom of my own. Thinking about that made me a little nervous but I knew that being a part of the staff at Deer Creek was going to be an amazing experience. I was excited to see what this new chapter of my life would bring.

It didn't take long for me to realize how blessed I was to work at Deer Creek Elementary. When I accepted the job at Deer Creek, I had no idea how many amazing people (staff and students) were about to come into my life. The staff quickly became a second family to me. I could not have asked to work with a better staff. During my first year of teaching, I had (and still do have) amazing support from the staff. To this day, I feel incredibly blessed to work with the staff and students of Deer Creek. I could not imagine being anywhere else.

During my first year of teaching, in March 2013, I ended up moving to Bailey. I lived with my parents in Conifer up until that point. Throughout the year, I was looking to see what was available to rent in the Conifer or Bailey area. When Aimee found out I was looking to move out of my parents' house, she brought up the idea of us being roommates. Aimee too wanted to move out of her parents' house and find a place within the mountain community. In

March 2013, we found the perfect place located less than ten minutes from Deer Creek. We both were so excited to move in and be a part of the Bailey community.

Within a short period, I realized how blessed I was to not only be teaching but also living within the Bailey community. I felt there definitely was a reason that my life's journey guided me to Bailey. I believe that you are meant to cross paths with certain people in your life. Without a doubt, there is a reason that the staff at Deer Creek came into my life. I'll forever be thankful for the close friendships I have developed while working there. Those close friends were the reason I was able to get through some challenging times. I could not imagine my life without the friends I have made at Deer Creek.

March 2016 was the first time I told anyone from work that I had a genetic disorder. During that month, I attended a training with the staff at Deer Creek called *Capturing Kids Hearts*. That training is where I first learned the definition of reframing. On day two of the training, the trainer showed us the definition of reframing and challenged us to think about a time we had reframed something. Immediately, I thought about my visits to the children's hospital. The words "negative comment or situation" in the definition made me think of different aspects of those hospital visits. I would definitely say that those visits to the hospital were some of the most negative situations I have had to deal with in my life. No one in particular made them negative situations. I thought of the visits as negative situations just because of the emotions that were involved with them. So many negative emotions went into those visits. I felt like I had been able to take those "negative situations" and "change my perspective on it," so I could move on.

After being told the definition of reframing, we were given time to think about when we had reframed a situation in our lives. Then we were told to find a partner and share our experiences with each other. When I was trying to find my partner, I honestly needed to remind myself again that I chose not to let Turner syndrome define me. The partner that I was about to sit down and talk with would be the first person at work to find out about me having a genetic disorder. I found a partner, and we went somewhere we could talk privately. As we sat down, I volunteered to share my experience first. I took a deep breath and began to talk. I didn't tell her the entire story but explained that I had a genetic disorder, and how I had to "reframe" a visit to the children's hospital. In the end, my coworker and I had a great talk. Just like my friends, my coworker reacted to the news in a positive way. I don't remember if I ever told her the name of my genetic disorder, but I was surprised I was able to share as much as I did. At that time, I did not know it, but I was two years away from being at a place in my life where I'd find the courage to open up to more friends from work.

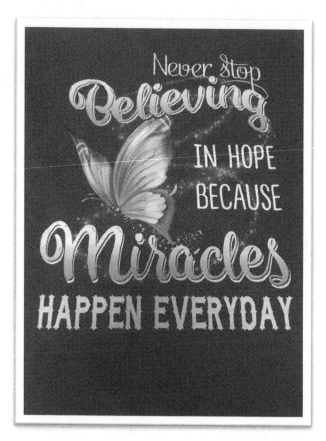

(Photograph of a t-shirt that was given to me as a gift)

CHAPTER 8

Taking Down Barriers

Just as my life took an unexpected turn when I was sixteen, it took another one when I was twenty-seven. December 29, 2017 was when this unexpected turn happened. On that day, per my primary care physician's recommendation, I had an appointment with an obstetrician-gynecologist (OB-GYN). It was recommended that I have the appointment to discuss the medication I was on and any other concerns I had. Even though I knew about the appointment for months, it didn't make it any easier for me. I woke up on that December day, and my anxiety hit me like a ton of bricks. Looking back, I am surprised I was actually able to get myself in the car. The drive to the appointment was full of tears. The entire time, I prayed for the strength and courage to get through the appointment. I desperately wanted to remain calm but doctor's appointments always triggered my anxiety. Forty minutes later, I was parked and walking into the appointment.

At that appointment, I found out that I needed to follow up with another specialist. The doctor I saw was extremely kind and easily determined that I was anxious. I was thankful that she was the doctor who saw me because she understood my anxiety and helped calm me down. I left that day knowing that I needed to make an appointment with another specialist during my spring or summer break. Walking out the door, I had mixed emotions. Overall, I felt my prayers for strength and courage had been answered. I did manage to make it through that appointment. I was anxious about having to schedule the appointment with the other specialist though. It was hard for me to fully grasp my feelings about that appointment as I drove home.

On that day, I didn't know it, but that appointment was the beginning of yet another journey for me. Following that appointment, a lot happened in my life. In the month of January 2018, I knew when the appointment with the specialist was tentatively going to be. At that point, I determined it was probably time to tell Thomas, the person I was dating, about me having Turner syndrome. Telling Thomas would be the first time I ever told someone I was dating about my condition. I'd be lying if I said I wasn't scared to tell him. So much was going through my mind before I told him. At the age of sixteen when I found out about having Turner syndrome, I was never given a guidebook on how to talk to someone I was dating about my condition. I had no idea how to start the conversation. In addition, I had no idea what kind of reaction I was going to get from Thomas when I told him.

The day that I told Thomas about my condition, we ended up talking for two hours. To be completely honest, I didn't tell him the name of my condition during that initial conversation. I told him about the condition and what it meant.

I went into all the details about how it would affect the future. In that particular moment, it was more important for me to explain what the condition meant for my future (especially with pregnancies) than stating the name. Overall, I felt the conversation went as well as I could have imagined. I knew that it was a lot of information for Thomas to process, and I respected that. It felt nice to finally have the information known and out in the open.

In the end, I was glad Thomas and I talked. Having that first conversation, opened the door to more communication about my diagnosis and helped our relationship grow. From that point on, we were able to have more conversations and really talk everything through. The conversations weren't always easy, but they led to positive outcomes. Once we started having conversations, Thomas worked to ensure me that he would be a support system.

Within a short time, I told two teachers and close friends at Deer Creek about me having Turner syndrome. I told Tina (a kindergarten teacher) and Maurita (another special education teacher).

Tina and Maurita are two people who I am incredibly blessed to know and call my friends. I told them both at separate times when I felt the time was right. There were defining moments when I just knew it was right for me to tell them.

I'll never forget the conversation I had with Tina when I told her I had Turner syndrome. It happened one day after school. Prior to our conversation that day, Tina knew I had a genetic disorder. I had told her in a previous conversation that I had a genetic disorder, but I never told her the name of it or anything about it. That day after school, we ended up staying in her classroom and talking for a couple of hours. Initially, I had gone into her classroom to check on her because I knew it had been a rough afternoon. I wanted to make sure that she was ok. We started talking and completely lost track of time. Eventually, we started walking towards the front of the building, so that Tina could do a couple things before an event at the school started. That evening, there was an event for the parents of incoming kindergarten students. As we were walking, something inside me told me it was the right time to open up to her about my condition. I felt the urge to talk to her about it. That night, standing outside of my office room, I told her about everything. I told her about the doctor's appointment when I was sixteen, that I had Turner syndrome, and some information about what it meant. Walking out of the school building that night, I couldn't have been happier that I had told Tina everything. She was someone I completely trusted, and it felt like some weight had been lifted off my shoulders.

Just as I knew when the time was right for me to tell Tina about my condition, I knew when the time was right to tell Maurita too. I told Maurita in her classroom one day when we were talking about doctor's appointments and health insurance. At that point, I knew I would have to see a specialist over spring or summer break. Due to the context of our conversation, it was fairly easy to bring everything up. Once I told her that I had to make an appointment with a specialist, the rest of the information just came out. I explained that I had Turner syndrome, what it meant, and why I had to go to a specialist. Again, it felt good for me to open up to someone else. At that point, I had known

Maurita for over five years. I was happy that I had finally been able to share that personal information with her.

With my upcoming doctor's appointment, I was incredibly thankful that I had told Tina and Maurita about my condition. They both were extremely supportive. Also, it was relieving to finally have people at work know about it. After telling Maurita and Tina, I was faced with some difficult emotional times. Certain things would trigger my anxiety about my upcoming doctor's appointment. Tina and Maurita both gave me incredible advice throughout everything, and I learned some amazing lessons from them.

After I told Tina about me having Turner syndrome, we had more conversations about it. I turned to her when those triggers that caused anxiety occurred. I was honest with her about conversations people had with me that triggered anxiety. When I say that conversations were a trigger, I know that it was not intentional by any means. However, there were things brought up in conversation that triggered my anxiety. Also, during the month of March 2018 (the month my appointment was scheduled), I was honest with Tina about the fact that March (in itself) was a trigger. I opened up to Tina about a lot throughout those months.

Not only did I open up to Tina in moments when I felt anxious, I also shared with her my moments of personal victory. Once I opened up to Tina, there were (without a doubt) moments of anxiety, but there were also moments of personal victories within my journey. I was always excited to share those stories with Tina.

One of my personal victories was when I opened up to my mom about what happened the day I found out I have Turner syndrome. My mom and I talk frequently on the phone. I call her every morning before school, and we generally talk each evening. One evening, in the beginning of March, I was talking with my mom on the phone and my upcoming doctor's appointment was brought up. I explained that I had been given the opportunity to have a brief phone conversation with the specialist who I would be meeting with at the end of the month. She asked what we had talked about, and I gave her a brief summary of what we discussed. I said that I was hopeful that the conversation I had with the specialist and being honest about my anxiety towards the appointment would help me. At that point, my mom asked me why I was so anxious. In that moment, I didn't know exactly what to say. I did not know if my mom knew what had happened at the doctor's appointment when I was sixteen. After thinking about it for a little bit, I told her that my anxiety really stemmed from the doctor's appointment in which I found out I have Turner syndrome. She then asked for more clarification on what happened at that appointment. I ended up asking her what she remembered about that day. Her answer told me what I needed to do next. She clearly did not know the full story regarding the appointment. She did not know that I overheard my dad tell the doctor I have Turner syndrome. I took a deep breath and told her there was more to the story. I then explained everything.

Having that conversation with my mom was a personal victory for me. I spent twelve years without knowing if she knew what had happened at that doctor's appointment when I was sixteen. I honestly thought that she had figured out what had happened on her own. I thought me coming out and asking if I had Turner syndrome after that specific appointment was indication that I found out somehow. Twelve years later, though, she finally knew everything. That conversation with my mom brought a mix of emotions. I was scared because, deep down, I didn't want my mom to be hurt or upset about what I told her. I was also relieved because the story was finally common knowledge between us. I no longer had to question if my mom knew how I found out about my diagnosis. Not having to question that anymore was a personal victory in itself.

The next day at school, I told Tina about the conversation I had with the specialist and my mother. I appreciated how she was always there to listen and provide support when needed. I enjoyed sharing stories with her along the journey. Every time I had another personal victory, I told her. Throughout the conversations that I had with Tina, she taught me a lot. Tina helped me realize that I had a lot of strength within me.

Maurita also taught me a lot through conversations I had with her. I think one of the most important lessons that Maurita taught me was about emotions and attaching them to things or experiences. One day, when we were having a conversation about my upcoming doctor's appointment, she told me I had the choice on which emotion I was attaching to it. It was clear that I was attaching anxiety to it. Every time I thought of going to the specialist, I was brought back to the appointment I had when I was sixteen, which triggered lots of anxiety. Maurita taught me to think about my emotions and the power I have. Of course, it is much easier to say, "I'm no longer going to attach anxiety to doctor's appointments" than actually doing it. I knew it was going to be hard not to attach anxiety to my upcoming appointment. I spent time reflecting on what Maurita had told me and realized there was truth to it. It is true that we have the power to decide what emotions we are attaching to something. When we attach an emotion to something, we can decide if it is going to be positive or negative. After that conversation with Maurita, I tried to be very mindful of the emotions I was attaching to my upcoming appointment.

Once I had told Tina and Maurita about me having Turner syndrome, it was easier for me to open the doors of communication with others. Before I knew it, I had opened up to other important people about my condition. Three very important people to me — Kay, Terri, and Clare — were the next colleagues from school that I had conversations with. After I told them all, I realized that I had an incredible support system surrounding me. The conversations that I had with each of them made me realize how lucky I was to have them all in my life. As I was mentally preparing myself for my upcoming doctor's appointment, it felt amazing to know I had so many important people in my life supporting me. Within a short time, I had increased the number of people I could turn to for support and words can't describe what that felt like. I guess it felt like I had finally decided I was no longer going to live with a secret. I decided I was done not talking about me having

Turner syndrome with other people. Making those decisions was an adrenaline rush. It was such a positive feeling.

As the doctor's appointment approached, there were people who offered to go with me for emotional support. The fact that those people offered to go and support me meant a lot. It made me further realize just how strong the support system I had was. Getting those offers made me think a lot about what would be best for me. I was constantly asking myself if I should go to the appointment by myself or if I should take someone with me. A phone conversation I had one day helped me figure out what decision I needed to make for myself.

This phone conversation was with Terri. She is someone who I have been blessed to know since I graduated from college. I first met Terri when I started working at Deer Creek Elementary. At the time, she was the District Psychologist. After my first year of teaching, she transitioned to the position of Executive Director for the Mt Evans BOCES. My district is within the Mt. Evans BOCES, so I continued to work closely with

Terri. Throughout the years, I have come to know Terri as not only a professional I can look up to but also an all-around great person. One day, before spring break in March 2018, something within me guided me to call her.

The week before spring break, there was one day in particular when my anxiety hit me pretty hard. I think I was in shock that it already was time for spring break. It felt like I had made the appointment with the specialist only yesterday. I couldn't believe it was coming up so quickly. That particular day, I also found out that Tina would most likely be moving in the beginning of April. The news of Tina moving, of course, made me sad. I couldn't imagine Deer Creek without her. After school that day, as I was walking to my car, our school counselor Breeann gave me some advice. She knew that it had been a rough day for me. As we walked to our cars, she asked if there was anything she could do for me. In that moment, I could not think of anything. I was trying to grasp the fact that my doctor's appointment was in a short time and Tina would be leaving soon too. Processing that information was hard for me. Thinking of both of those events stirred up many emotions. When I told Breeann that I couldn't think of anything I needed, she gave me a hug and said that if I ever needed to talk, she was there for me. She also told me that I should go home and call someone to talk to. It didn't matter who it was, but she said that talking with someone would probably be good for me. Immediately, Terri came to my mind. I got in my car, drove home, and called Terri.

That night, Terri talked with me for over forty minutes. I ended up telling her about me having Turner syndrome during that phone call. Just like Tina and Maurita had taught me a lot, I took away some lessons from my conversation with Terri. Terri helped me reflect on what was causing me to be so anxious and what steps I needed to take for myself. When I was talking with Terri, I had so much going through my mind. I told her I was trying to determine what would be best for me as far as taking someone to the appointment or going alone. I also said that I was a little nervous about how I would act the day of the appointment due to my anxiety. I explained that I didn't know if I wanted someone going to the appointment with me because of that reason. Terri listened and was able to talk me through a lot. In the end, I was very glad that I had picked up the phone to call her. At the end of the conversation, I felt like I had more clarity on the next steps I should take. I was thankful that Breeann had given me the advice to call someone.

Honestly, it did make me a little nervous to make the call to Terri. The fact that I was nervous had nothing to do with her as a person. I was nervous because I knew I would most likely tell her a lot of personal information during the conversation. After talking with her though, I felt a lot better. Not only did I feel better, I knew I had added her to the list of people who I could turn to for support. Having her in that group of people meant a lot to me. I was happy that I had made the decision to call her. There definitely is a reason that I was guided to call her that night.

Before I knew it, spring break had arrived. Normally, I would have been really excited to have a week off. To be honest though, this time I started spring break feeling more anxious than excited. I would have been all right with still being at school. My appointment with the specialist wasn't until later in the week. It would have been easy for me to spend all the time leading up to my appointment at home doing nothing. At the start of spring break, I decided I was not going to let myself do that though. I wanted to make the best of my time off and spend it with people I cared about. I made plans with friends and did not let myself stay home much.

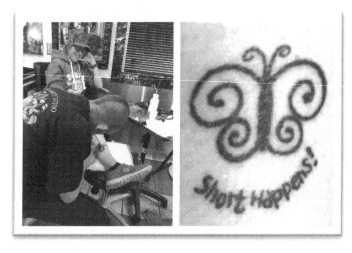

*(**Left Photo**: Me getting my tattoo in March 2018*
Right Photo: *Tattoo done by Charles Downey at*
Celebrity Tattoo in Lakewood, Colorado)

CHAPTER 9

Inked

Prior to spring break, I was doing some random Internet searches on Turner syndrome. While doing my research, something made me think of awareness ribbons and symbols that represent various medical conditions. I cannot tell you what made me think of it but something did. I thought of the Down Syndrome awareness ribbon my sister had tattooed on her foot. Immediately, I typed "Turner syndrome Awareness" on Google. The search came up with a purple awareness ribbon and an awareness symbol. The symbol was of a butterfly with the words "Short Happens!" underneath it.

That Google search inspired me to do some more research on the butterfly. Upon doing more research, I found out that the butterfly had become a symbol for girls with Turner syndrome because butterflies are considered fragile and beautiful miracles. I also found out that the particular butterfly I saw with the words "Short Happens!" underneath it was a symbol for the Turner Syndrome Society of the United States. After doing the research, I immediately thought of getting it as a tattoo. I thought it could be a symbol to remind me to empower myself. The first Saturday of spring break, I found myself looking at the symbol once again and seriously considering the tattoo.

That same night, I went to a Mammoth game with my friend Aimee. I met her at her grandmother's house before the game. Prior to the game, we took her dog for a walk in a nearby park. As we were walking, I told Aimee that I had possibly found something I wanted tattooed on me. She chuckled and then asked what my idea was. I pulled out my phone, showed her the picture of the awareness symbol, and explained what it was. She immediately loved the idea of me getting that particular tattoo. I told her I was seriously considering it but didn't know when I would get it. I chuckled and told her something along the lines of, "Depending on what direction my life takes after the doctor's appointment, maybe I will get it." We continued walking and discussing my upcoming appointment. Aimee once again offered to go the appointment with me if I wanted her too. As we were walking, I was so glad that I had Aimee in my life. It was crazy for me to think that we were going on eighteen years of friendship. She is definitely a friend I am blessed to have. I was looking forward to spending the evening at the Mammoth game with her.

The morning after the Mammoth game, I woke up with the urge to get the tattoo. I know that just the day before I had said that I wasn't going to get it until after the appointment, but I changed my mind that morning. After thinking about it, I thought getting it before the appointment would help me empower myself for it. I got up, dressed, and got in my car. I decided that I was driving either to go grocery shopping or to go get the tattoo and then go shopping. Either way, I knew I was leaving the house. I drove to the grocery store and sat in the parking lot. On my phone, I did some research on tattoo parlors nearby. I found one that had good reviews and called them. I called to see if they were open and asked if I could come in without an appointment. Once they told me I didn't need an appointment, I called Aimee. When she answered, she was driving home from breakfast with her boyfriend. I told her that I was seriously considering driving down to the tattoo parlor. It turned out that the tattoo parlor I was considering was the same one Aimee had got her tattoos at. Aimee agreed to meet me if I decided to go. Next thing I knew, I was driving down to Celebrity Tattoo in Lakewood, Colorado.

When I arrived at the tattoo parlor, I was in complete shock that I was actually considering a tattoo. People who know me really well would probably say I'm the last person they would expect to get a tattoo because of my needle phobia. I could not believe that I was about to walk into a tattoo parlor and actually get one. Walking into the building with Aimee, I was afraid that I was going to change my mind. I was a little anxious about how much it would hurt. I didn't know if I actually would go through with it.

We walked in the building and talked with Charles, one of the tattoo artists. I showed him a picture of the awareness symbol, and he said it would be easy for him to do. He also assured me that it would not hurt as much as I thought. I filled out the paperwork and next thing I knew, he was bringing me a stencil of the tattoo. At that point, it was time to put the stencil on and start with the tattoo. Aimee and I followed him back to his chair, and I sat down. He put the stencil on my leg and had me look in a mirror to see if I liked how it looked. After agreeing on the placement and the size, I sat back down and braced myself for what was next. Charles picked up his tattoo gun and began working. Aimee started taking pictures on my phone, so we had proof I actually got a tattoo.

After Aimee had taken some pictures, I asked her for my phone so I could text one to my sister. I knew my sister would be in shock when she found out I was getting a tattoo. I sent her a picture of me sitting in the chair, and the tattoo artist working on the tattoo. The caption I sent with the picture was, "So this is happening..." In less than two minutes, I received, "WHAT?!? What are you getting?!?! Who are you with? Where are you?" from her. At that point, I didn't know how to answer my sister's question about what tattoo I was getting. I honestly had never had a conversation with my sister about me having Turner syndrome. I didn't even know if she knew about it. I sent her a message back saying that I was getting an awareness symbol for the genetic disorder I had a form of. I explained it was a symbol with some text underneath it. Immediately, my sister sent me a picture of the awareness symbol with the text, "This one?" I was shocked at how quickly she sent me the picture. I had shown the exact same picture to the tattoo artist. The tattoo wasn't even completely done, and already it was helping me open up doors of communication. My sister and I had our first conversation about it.

When I had my first look at the completed tattoo, I fell in love with it. It looked absolutely perfect. I could not believe I actually had gone through with it. In the end, the pain wasn't as bad as I thought it was going to be. Looking at the completed product, I felt so empowered. Getting the tattoo was a way for me to prove to myself that I could get through something that caused anxiety. Words can't describe how empowered I felt after getting the tattoo. I walked out of the tattoo parlor extremely happy that I had a permanent symbol of empowerment I could look at whenever I wanted. I was so thankful that Aimee went with me on such short notice that day. She was the perfect friend to take on that adventure. As I walked out of the tattoo parlor, the tattoo artist and Aimee both told me it would only be a matter of time until I got another. I didn't want to believe them, but I knew they were right.

Once I got in my car, I called my mom to tell her I got the tattoo. She knew I had been considering it but didn't know I actually went through with it that day. When I told her, she was shocked. She wanted picture proof to show that I had actually gone through with it. I think she is still in shock that I went through with it. I know she never expected me to actually get a tattoo. We continued talking, and I ended up asking her a question that I had been thinking about for many years. I asked her if our extended family knew about me having Turner syndrome. I specifically wanted to know if my Aunt JoAnn and Aunt Dawn knew about it. She told me that they both have known since I was born.

The fact that my Aunts had known about my diagnosis since my birth could easily have stirred up some anger. For a brief period, I did think to myself, "I didn't find out the name to my condition until I was sixteen, and members of my extended family have known since I was born!" It would have been easy for me to be angry about that. In the end though, I didn't let those emotions consume me. I decided I was focusing on the present moment. At that moment, I found out that my extended family knew about my condition, and I chose to use that knowledge to open doors of communication. There was no point in dwelling on the past because it had already happened.

Instead of focusing on the exact time that my extended family had found out about my condition, I found comfort in the fact that they knew about it.

The same day that I got my tattoo, I called both my Aunt JoAnn and Aunt Dawn. I was excited to tell them about it because I was sure they would be shocked like my mom. Aunt JoAnn was the first one I got in touch with. When I told her I got a tattoo, she definitely was shocked. I remember after I told her she said, "You got a what?" Then I repeated myself and she said, "That's what I thought you said. WOW!" I then went on to explain what the tattoo was and what it meant. She, of course, immediately wanted a picture sent to her too. That conversation with my Aunt JoAnn was the first time I ever talked to her about me having Turner syndrome. Through that conversation, I felt that I had opened up yet another door of communication.

After talking with my Aunt JoAnn, I was able to talk with my cousin, Ginger, too. Near the end of our conversation, my Aunt JoAnn said, "I'm going to hand the phone to your cousin, so you can tell her what you did today. I don't think she would believe me if I told her." Ginger and I ended up talking for about fifteen minutes or so that day. We are separated by four years, but I feel I have always had a close bond with her. I was excited to tell her about my tattoo. When I was telling her about it, she told me she knew I had been born with a genetic disorder. She loved the fact that I got a tattoo that was so symbolic and meant something to me. I was glad I had the opportunity to talk with Ginger that day.

When I talked with my Aunt Dawn, she also was surprised that I got a tattoo but really excited about it. I had sent her a text with a picture of it, so she had already seen it. When I explained the meaning behind the tattoo, she told me that she knew I was born with a genetic disorder, but that she didn't remember its name. Hearing her say that actually made me realize that while my extended family knew about it, they didn't make a big deal of it. It made me feel pretty good. Within a short time, I had talked with three extended family members about my condition for the first time. It felt like even more weight was lifted off my shoulders.

(Tattoo done by Charles Downey at Celebrity Tattoo in Lakewood, Colorado)

CHAPTER 10

The Appointment

The rest of my spring break, leading up to my appointment, was spent doing fun things with friends. As I said before, I wasn't going to let myself just sit at home even though that would have been easy to do. I went to the movies with Kelsey Poole, went on a double date, and even took a trip up to Greeley (the town I graduated college from) with my mom to see my friend Lance. Overall, I found myself enjoying spring break. It was great to spend time with friends and get out of the house. It definitely made spring break a lot more enjoyable and helped me not to dwell on my anxiety. I think being out of the house actually helped reduce my anxiety.

Wednesday night (the day before my appointment), I had a phone conversation with Tina. By Wednesday night, I was pretty certain that I wanted Tina to be the one to go to the appointment with me. I knew I was at a place where I could probably handle talking with the doctor on my own, but I thought it would be good to have her there. I felt there would be a sense of comfort to know I could have her by my side at any time during the appointment, if needed. We talked on the phone that night so that we could finalize plans for the next day.

That night, Tina said something that really resonated with me and caused me to reflect a lot. I told her that I was a little nervous about how I was going to be feeling in the morning. I thought back to my appointment in December 2017 when I was so anxious and crying the whole drive to it. At that point, Tina pointed out how far I had come since that appointment. She went on to say that I had pretty much been running a race for years that not many people knew about.

Since December 2017, she had watched me take down barriers and let people in. She said I now had more people on the sidelines cheering for me because I took down those barriers. Tina gave me a perspective that I had never thought about before. I never would have compared the journey I was on to running a race and taking down barriers. Upon reflecting though, it made complete sense to me. Those words were exactly what I needed to hear that night. Those words helped me realize how much power and strength I had within myself.

On the day of my appointment, I woke up feeling anxious but doing better than I thought I would be. I started my day and got myself ready. Before I left the house, I spent some time praying. I put on one of my favorite spiritual songs and prayed as I listened. I prayed for the strength, courage, and guidance I needed to get through the day. Praying helped me to get in the right mindset to face the day. At 11:00 a.m., I left to go and pick Tina up from her house.

The whole ride down to the doctor's appointment, we listened to *The Greatest*

Showman soundtrack (music that we both really enjoy) and talked. We talked about the doctor's appointment and many other things. As we were driving to the appointment, I constantly thought of how thankful I was to have Tina with me. Having her with me kept me calm on the drive down the mountain and I knew it would help me once we got to the appointment. It became clear to me that I had made the right choice to have her with me.

As I pulled into the parking lot of the medical building, I felt my stomach drop a little. My anxiety was definitely kicking in. Tina and I sat in my car for a little bit before going into the building. When I had fifteen minutes remaining until my appointment, we made our way into the building. I was nervous but having her with me made it easier. We made our way to the appropriate office within the medical building. Within minutes, I was signed in for the appointment and filling out a mountain of new patient paperwork.

It wasn't long after filling out the paperwork that I was called in to meet with the doctor. As usual, my vitals were taken first, and then I was escorted to the room that my doctor was in. When I was taken into the room, I was actually surprised. As I entered the room, I saw the doctor, dressed in business casual clothes, sitting behind a desk. It was not your typical doctor's examination room. I shook the doctor's hand, introduced myself, and sat down in a chair in front of the desk. Most of my appointment was spent in that room. We had lengthy discussions about the medication I was on, my health history, and the testing done at the children's hospital. When it came to my medication, we discussed the different options I had. For twelve years, I had been on a medication called Estradiol as a form of hormone replacement therapy. My doctor and I discussed increasing the dose of Estradiol and adding another medication to my routine. She explained some possible side effects of the medication and what to do if I had them. In the end, I agreed to move forward with the medication changes. As we were talking about the medication, I realized how great it felt to be in charge of making the decisions. The doctor discussed everything with me and took my input on what the next steps should be. Getting to make the decisions was so empowering in itself.

After talking for a little bit, she said that she wanted to move to an examination room to do a brief physical examination. Those words instantly made me a little nervous. I asked her what the examination would entail. After talking it through, I followed her into the examination room next door. She completed the physical exam pretty quickly and then took me back into her office room, so we could finish the appointment. Right after we got back in her office, I saw my cell phone screen (which was sitting on the chair next to me) light up. I quickly glanced to see a message from Kay that said, "Thinking of you! Hope it is all going well." At that moment, I smiled, took a deep breath, and felt calm. Her message reminded me of how thankful I am to have her in my life. At that point, I knew the end of the appointment was approaching, and that I could handle it.

We finished the appointment by discussing the next steps. The doctor explained that there were things she wanted me to follow up on as precautionary measures. It wasn't that she thought something was wrong; it was just that it was time to monitor specific things again. Overall, I handled that aspect of the appointment so much better than I thought I would. I had prepared myself for the possibility of follow up tests. I guess I saw it coming. As my appointment was ending, I developed a timeline with my doctor of when those things would be taken care of. The timeline helped me to process everything and know what to expect. This time around, as opposed to when I was sixteen, I felt like I had more control. That made things easier for me to handle. I was given a lot of paperwork to take with me and then the appointment was over. As I departed my doctor's office, I had a pretty good impression of her.

I walked out to the waiting room, gave the front desk some of the paperwork, and then sat next to Tina. I had no idea what to say at that moment. I think I just looked at Tina and said with a smile, "I did it; it's done!" As we walked out the building, I told her I would probably talk her ear off when we got back in the car. I wanted to tell her everything that had just happened. I knew that talking about it would help me sort out all the information that had been discussed. We sat in my car and talked for about ten minutes before leaving. I felt I needed to talk a little bit before driving. After talking for a while, we decided to go out to lunch before heading back to Bailey.

At lunch, I was able to talk to Tina a little more about what the doctor had said. I was glad that we had decided to go out to eat. It was nice to have some more time to just sit and talk. When we were eating lunch, I realized again how lucky I was to have Tina in my life. I know I would not have been able to get through the day if it wasn't for her. It meant so much that Tina had given her day to come and support me. I knew she was in the process of trying to get things done before moving, but she still came anyway. I was so thankful for her support that day.

In the end, I knew that taking Tina to the appointment with me was the right decision. I know that my mom would have taken the day off to come with me in a heartbeat. We had a couple different conversations about that. When it was brought up, I always thanked my mom for her willingness to go with me. Each time we discussed it, I told her that I appreciated the offer to go to the appointment, but then explained I was trying to determine what was best for me. I explained that I actually didn't know if I was going to take anyone with me at all. I also said that if I decided I wanted someone to go with me, I would probably be taking a friend. Admitting that I would take a friend with me to the appointment was hard because I didn't want to hurt my mom. I was completely honest with her though and told her that it may be better for someone other than a family member to be with me. I felt that taking someone else would force me to keep calm.

Whenever my mom and I had a conversation about the upcoming doctor's appointment, I assured her that the friend I'd pick to go with me was someone who knew about my condition. I told her I had been frequently talking with Tina about everything. I like to think that assuring my mom of that helped her feel comfortable with my decision. I appreciated how supportive my mom was of the decisions I made regarding the doctor's appointment. Not once did she pressure me to come along. Not once did she question my thoughts about it. It made me feel so much better about the entire situation. Tina had a calming effect on me the day of my appointment, which is exactly what I needed. Without a doubt, I made the right decision for myself that day. I was happy that I had the courage to make the choice that was best for me.

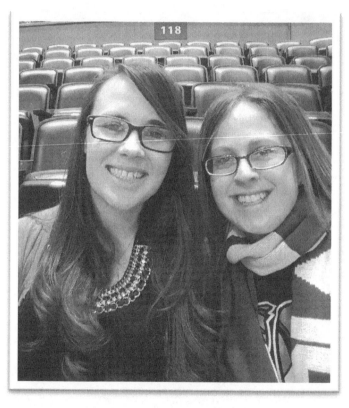

(Aimee and me at a Colorado Mammoth game during the 2018 season)

CHAPTER 11

Surrounded by an Amazing Tribe

The day after my doctor's appointment, I woke up not feeling too good. Before I had gone to bed the previous night, I started my new medication routine. Immediately after waking up, I could feel some of the side effects my doctor told me about. I felt drowsy and nauseous—two things that are not fun combined. I attempted to eat some breakfast to see if that would help me. A couple hours after breakfast, there wasn't much difference in how I felt. At that point, I didn't know what to do. I considered calling or emailing my doctor but then decided that maybe my body was just adjusting to the medication. I pulled out my paperwork from the doctor to read some more about the medication and to determine what I should do. While I was looking through the paperwork, it dawned on me that I had a resource I could turn to within my family. I picked up my phone and called my Aunt JoAnn.

My Aunt JoAnn has been through nursing school and worked as a nurse in a hospital. For medical reasons, she is not currently a practicing nurse, but she does still work in a hospital. I thought she would be a good person to call and talk about my medications. As I dialed her number, I was 100 percent comfortable calling her because of the conversation we had the day I got my tattoo. That conversation made it clear to me that she knew about me having Turner syndrome. Since we had that conversation, the door of communication was open. I had no problems with calling to ask her about the medications.

Talking with my Aunt validated what I had been thinking. She told me to give it some time before calling my doctor. I was right in my thinking that my body needed some time to adjust. She was able to help me decide how long I should wait before calling my doctor. Having the conversation with her made me feel better. It made me worry a little less. After having that conversation with my Aunt, I was able to relax the rest of the day. I'd be lying if I said I wasn't nervous to take the medication again that night, but I woke up the next day feeling better.

Finally, when spring break came to end, I realized it had been a pleasant week. Spending time doing things I enjoy with friends and family made such a huge difference. Getting out of the house helped me control my anxiety as my appointment approached. One important lesson I learned during the week was that it was powerful to surround yourself with those you care about.

While the side effects from my medication went away quickly, I felt a little more emotional than normal as my body was adjusting to the medication. Tina's last day at Deer Creek came the week after spring break. That day was definitely very emotional for me. I knew it was a "see you later" and not a "goodbye," but it was still very difficult for me to grasp. I got much more emotional than I thought I would. In an effort to try to process everything, I called my friend Cindy who had just gone through the same thing with a friend at work. A close work friend of Cindy's had recently moved out of the state just as Tina was. Cindy was able to help reassure me that everything was going to be ok. The night I called her, I knew what I needed to hear from her — that she was ok.

In the days that followed Tina's last day, I had so many incredible people supporting me. Terri, Kay, Maurita, and Clare were all there to provide support in whatever way I needed, which I was so thankful for. There was a brief period when I felt more emotional as my body adjusted to the medicine. I also had to step back and realize that I had gone through a lot within a short time. Preparing for and anticipating my doctor's appointment along with Tina's last day both stirred up some difficult emotions. Both events also happened close together. I think there were a couple of different factors that were making me emotional. The support I got during that time made everything so much easier to deal with. Clare spent a night at my house to talk with me. Her presence was calming. Maurita and Kay were there for me during school days when I felt emotional. Kay, who was previously our Assistant Principal but transitioned to District Assessment Coordinator, spent a lot of time at Deer Creek following spring break. She and Maurita were there to talk or do whatever they could to support me when things got tough during school days. Terri came to Deer Creek to support me through an IEP meeting and to help get some other things done. It meant so much to have them all by my side.

In the moments when I had people supporting me, I realized how incredibly lucky I was. I am a firm believer that everything happens for a reason. I also believe that there is a reason for everyone you meet. When I think back to everything that happened in my life from December 2017 to March 2018, I couldn't imagine doing it without the support of some incredible people. Finding the courage to open up to people at work was one of the best things that ever happened to me. Yes, I was extremely nervous to open up to those people. It was a huge risk. The result of taking that risk though was an amazing support system. I was able to build a support system that got me through so much. I'm so lucky to work with some amazing individuals that have quickly become like family.

The week after spring break, Aimee and I spent a lot of time talking on the phone. She would call to check on me, or I would call her to talk. One day, we ended up talking about everything that had happened in my life in the past three months. I don't remember how we got to that topic, or how the conversation even started. As I reflected though, I made a comment about how a lot had happened in my life, but I'd made some positive gains. Aimee then told me that it was as if I was finally embracing everything about my diagnosis and turning it into something positive. When I was sixteen, Aimee watched me go through everything as I found out about my diagnosis. Years later, she was watching me go through things again. To hear Aimee say that she noticed the positive changes in me was an incredible feeling. After that conversation, I thought about how I was truly starting to embrace everything. I realized that Aimee was right. I believed I was getting to a place in my life where I was allowing my condition to become part of my identity without shame. I'm blessed to have a friend that has been on this journey with me since day one.

That specific conversation with Aimee made me realize that I was not just embracing the fact that I have Turner syndrome, but also embracing the tribe of people surrounding me. When it comes down to it, I think the sixteen-year-old me was afraid to let people in on my journey for many reasons. Twelve years later, finally, letting go of that fear allowed me to fully embrace the support others wanted to give me. Fear no longer stood in the way of me talking about my condition to others or even openly expressing my emotions. I was finally allowing others to be a part of my journey and embracing their support. That support helped me more than I could ever say.

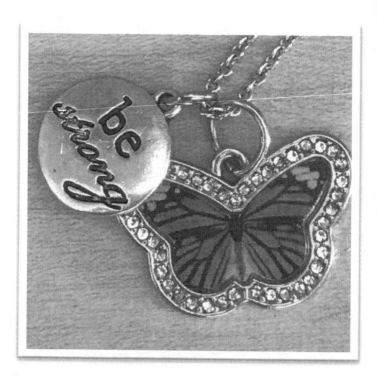

CHAPTER 12

Finding Strength

Leading up to my doctor's appointment (in March 2018) and even the week following it, there were times when I found myself in conversations about pregnancies and the options I had if I chose to have kids. I talked with Thomas, my mom, and other friends about it. I've always known that there are different options for women who can't have children naturally such as in-vitro fertilization, surrogacy, and even adoption. Since the day I found out I have Turner syndrome, I have been able to process that information and come to some conclusions about those options. However, I didn't talk a whole lot about it until I was twenty-eight. It was then that I realized I had come to a place in my life where I could openly talk about my thoughts regarding a future pregnancy. As I mentioned before, I have always wanted to be a mom someday. Nothing changes the fact that I want children, but I have been able to make some decisions on what I think would be the best way to achieve that. Being open and honest with everyone about my thoughts on the subject was a huge step for me. Some of the conversations were hard to have, but I was so glad I had them. It felt amazing to be open about my thoughts and not hold them in. At my doctor's appointment, we briefly talked about pregnancies and the different options. My doctor completely validated my feelings by saying it was ok for me to acknowledge the options that would be good for me and the ones that would not. She also reminded me that in the end, it was my decision on what I put my body through. At sixteen, I was definitely not ready to talk about (or even think about) the options. Over the course of twelve years though, I had come to a place in my journey where I was at peace with everything and could acknowledge which options I thought were best for me. I was happy to be at that place and openly discuss it. Once I started opening up to people in my life without holding back, it was such a liberating feeling.

It is safe to say that over a four-month period (December 2017 to March 2018); I had some difficult conversations with many people. Within that time, I had conversations with people about the fact that I have Turner syndrome, I opened up to my mom about the day I found out about my condition, I had conversations regarding my thoughts on pregnancies, conversations with my extended family for the first time, and conversations about my doctor's appointment. I remember, one day, being asked by a friend how I even started some of those conversations. After thinking about it, I really didn't know what to say. Some of the conversations I had within that short time were very difficult for me to initiate because of how nervous it made me. However, once I started having conversations with people, it made it much easier to continue opening up the doors of communication. Some of the conversations literally started with me taking a deep breath and telling myself, "I can do it." I didn't think a lot about the conversations; I just initiated them. Even though some of them were difficult to have, they were rewarding. I don't regret initiating any of the conversations. I learned through it all that even though some conversations can be nerve-wracking to have, so many positive things could come from them. It felt so much better to have those conversations than to hold everything in. I cannot imagine where I would be today if I hadn't taken the steps to open up to people about my condition. Initiating those conversations helped me get to a great place in my life.

As I reflect on the journey I have been on, I am thankful that I had the courage to open up to others and have some difficult conversations. At the age of sixteen, when I learned about my diagnosis, I did not open up to many people. As I mentioned earlier in my story, Aimee was the only friend who knew about my condition for a while. My parents and Aimee were the main people I talked to about everything I was going through. Twelve years later, I opened up to many more people about my condition. Going into my appointment with the specialist in March 2018 felt different. In March 2018, I walked into that appointment knowing there was an incredible group of supportive people who really cared about me. That fact in itself made a world of difference. It was almost as if I could physically feel the support from everyone as I went into the appointment. I learned that it is important to surround yourself with people you can always rely on for support. Even though it took me some time to be more open about my condition, I am grateful it happened. Being more open meant having some difficult conversations but it helped me become a stronger person.

I've heard people say that "being strong" means having the ability to go through a difficult time by yourself. I think there is a perception that asking for help or support makes someone weak. In 2018, it became clear to me how much strength it takes to be open and vulnerable. Today, I personally believe that opening up to people during difficult times takes a tremendous amount of strength. It took a lot of inner strength for me to be more open with others about my condition. Once I did open up to others, I learned that there is power in numbers. The bottom line is that the people I chose to surround myself with saw strength in me when it was difficult for me to see it myself. Knowing that they saw strength within me allowed me to become a stronger person. The more people I let in on my journey, the easier it was for me to find my strength. Without those people, I would not have seen so many positive gains in 2018. Strength is not about going through something alone. Strength is surrounding yourself with people who will show you just how strong you really are. The first four months of 2018 really made me reflect on what it means to "be strong." In addition, I learned just how strong I really was.

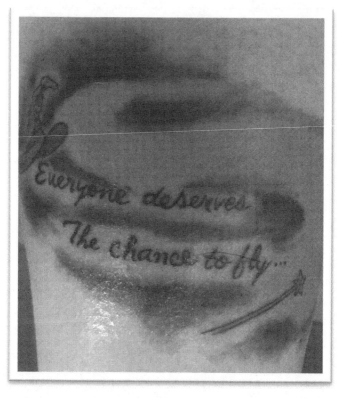

(Tattoo done by Charles Downey at Celebrity Tattoo in Lakewood, Colorado)

CHAPTER 13

Connected by Social Media

One day, in April 2018, as I was searching the Internet, I came across an interesting blog post. I was doing some research and found a blog post written by a woman with Turner syndrome. I read the blog post and realized I had some things in common with the woman who wrote it. The woman, like me, did not find out about her diagnosis until a little later in life. From the picture on the blog post, I guessed that we were both in our 20s. I also gathered that she lived in Colorado. After reading the blog post, I saw a link to a social media profile of hers. Once

I saw that link, I knew I had the choice to reach out to her if I wanted to. I opened up her profile and clicked on the button to send an email to her. For at least five minutes, I sat on my couch and stared at the screen.

In twenty-eight years, I had never talked to another woman or girl with Turner syndrome, and there I was with the opportunity. I had the opportunity to reach out to another woman, Ally, with my condition for the first time. I had no idea what to do. I had no idea what to say on my email. I stared at my screen contemplating what to do. I asked myself if I should email her or just let it go. Slowly, I started to type a message to her. In the message, I introduced myself, told her I have a form of Turner syndrome, and that I had read her blog. I also explained that I had never talked with another woman who has Turner syndrome but that reading her blog motivated me to send her an email. When I finished typing the message, I remember saying to myself that the past three months had been all about taking down barriers, so why not take down another one. I typed the message and hit the send button. I then eagerly waited to see if I would get a response.

Within a day, I had a response from Ally. We started sending messages back and forth, so we could get to know each other. I learned that she was twenty-two and was living in Littleton, which was not far from me. Talking with another woman who has Turner syndrome was such a surreal feeling. I can't even put words to it. I told Ally numerous times that I couldn't believe I was actually talking to someone else with Turner syndrome. She totally understood where I was coming from. Ally explained she felt the same way the first time she talked to someone else with Turner syndrome. On the first day that we started talking, we agreed that we wanted to continue sending messages to each other and even discussed meeting.

When I found out about having Turner syndrome, I can honestly say that I never expected to talk to another woman who has it. For some reason, that just wasn't a priority for me. It was something I never thought about. Twelve years after learning about my diagnosis, it was an incredible feeling to make that a priority. I think the decision to reach out to Ally was a sign of how much growth I had made. I truly was at a point in my life where I had made positive gains. I had taken down barriers. After realizing how far I had come, I wasn't going to let anything hold me back. If an opportunity to make even more positive gains presented itself, you bet I was going to take it.

That initial conversation I had with Ally presented some opportunities and inspired me to do some research. I learned through talking with Ally that there were organizations around the world devoted to helping women with Turner syndrome. Ally told me about Turner syndrome Colorado and the Turner syndrome Society of the United States. I quickly learned that the Turner Syndrome Society of the United States hosted a conference each summer. Ally told me she had attended it before and encouraged me to do some research on it. She also told me more about Turner Syndrome Colorado and how she has been involved with that organization. Prior to talking with Ally, I had not heard a lot about those specific organizations. I decided to do some research on both organizations to see what they were all about.

Over the course of a couple of days, I spent a lot of time researching the upcoming summer conference that would be hosted by the Turner Syndrome Society of the United States. I read about each of the seminars that would be offered and testimonies from other women who had attended the conference. In addition, I reached out to someone from Turner Syndrome Colorado. I thought that reaching out to someone in Colorado would help me make some decisions about the conference. By talking to Marybel, the founder of Turner Syndrome Colorado, I realized what steps I wanted to take next. I decided not going to the upcoming summer conference was best for me. The seminars offered at the conference were geared more towards the medical aspects of Turner syndrome. I realized that I was at a place in my life where I was seeking friendships and connections with other women who have my condition. Going to a conference to listen to medical seminars did not seem like the right step for me. I knew that I would obviously meet many women with my condition at the conference but didn't think that was the best setting for me to make those connections. The more I researched and thought about the conference, the more I realized that it could potentially trigger anxiety in me. When I spoke with Marybel, I was honest about what I was thinking and looking for. Marybel was supportive of everything I said and offered to help me in any way she could. She offered to reach out to some other women with Turner syndrome from Colorado, and see if they would be willing to talk with me. Even though I determined that attending the upcoming conference was not for me, I'm glad I took the time to research it. Throughout the time that I did research on the conference, I spent a lot of time reflecting on what was best for me. In the end, I knew that I was the only one who could make that decision. Knowledge is power, so I used what I learned about the conference to make the best decision for me. After absorbing all the information I found, I listened to my gut feeling about what steps I should take next. I knew that my primary focus should be on making connections with other women who have Turner syndrome outside of a conference setting. That is where I began to focus my energy. Once I had made decisions, it led to more doors being opened. Within a short time, I took a step that gave me the opportunity to be connected to many women with Turner syndrome.

It is almost mind blowing to think that social media was the way I talked to another woman with Turner syndrome for the first time. The world of social media has grown so much since it first emerged. I remember when I was in high school and MySpace was established. Within a short time, it seemed like everyone had his or her own MySpace page. Not too long after MySpace came Facebook. Today, there are numerous social media websites for people to choose from. I've always believed that social media comes with its pros and cons. When I first created a profile on Facebook, I enjoyed the fact that it allowed me to keep in close contact with friends and family. I especially liked it as a way to keep in contact with individuals out of state. Facebook made it easy to keep in touch with friends and family that didn't live close. I never imagined that social media would not only connect me to Ally one day but also connect me with literally thousands of other individuals with Turner syndrome.

A couple of weeks after I was connected with Ally, I typed "Turner syndrome" in the search bar on Facebook. That search showed me there were Facebook groups dedicated to women who have Turner syndrome and their families. The groups were private, which meant that I would have to send a request in order to join any of them. Once I found out about the Turner syndrome Facebook groups, I contemplated if I wanted to join one of them or not. I was already part of a Facebook group for the mountain community I live in. That group page is also private, and it is a way for members of the community to keep in contact. Members of the community use the group page to post local news or announcements among many other things. I spent time trying to decide if joining one of the Turner syndrome groups would be good for me or not. Eventually, I ended up sending a request to join one of the groups.

Once I joined the group, I spent some time reading the posts that individuals put on the page. As I read through posts and people's comments, it seemed like a group comprised of supportive women. I also saw that the group was made up of over 3000 people. Seeing that number made me ask myself, "I wonder how many of those women have Mosaic Tuner syndrome like me," and "I wonder how many of those women are teachers?" I had a desire to know more. After spending a lot of time reading the posts, I decided to write something of my own. I wrote a brief introduction to myself and posted it. Within minutes, I had responses. I had women from all over the world respond to me. Women who were in their 20s, women who were in the field of special education, and women who had Mosaic Turner syndrome were among the people who wrote back to me. Going through the comments on my post was a bizarre experience for me. It was crazy to think that social media had connected me with so many women who have Turner syndrome. In addition, social media also made me realize a lot about Turner syndrome. Joining that Facebook group showed me there were many women (around my age) who have the same form of the condition as I do. I also learned there were many women with Turner syndrome who were teachers. In addition, there were women in the group who had not learned about their diagnosis until later in life like me.

Over the course of a couple of days, I continued to read all the posts on the Facebook group. Numerous posts started with, "Hi, Turner syndrome sisters…" or "Hi, Turner syndrome Butterflies…." As I read the posts, I remember thinking to myself how cool it was that this group of women called themselves sisters and butterflies. I loved seeing how supportive they were of each other. It then hit me that being a part of the large group of women with Turner syndrome meant more than I thought. I learned that being a part of that group was way beyond just having the same medical condition. The women in the group seemed to share a bond that is like a sisterhood. I then realized that I was embracing being a Turner syndrome butterfly. Being a Turner syndrome butterfly meant I was part of a great group of women, and I was proud of that.

I'm glad that I decided to join the Facebook group. If I had discovered that group even four months earlier, I probably would not have joined it. When I did decide to join the group, I felt like I was finally at a place in my life where being a part of it made sense. I wanted to have connections with other women who have my condition. I figured joining the group would help me make those connections. After joining the group, I quickly realized that it felt amazing to have a way to connect with other women who have Turner syndrome.

Joining the Facebook group and writing a self-introduction lead to some good conversations with other women. I started emailing other women who were my age and have Mosaic Turner syndrome. I also started talking to other women within Colorado who have Turner syndrome. It was an eye opening experience for me when I finally had the connections I'd been seeking. It was incredible to know that within seconds, I could communicate with other women who have the same condition as me. It was fun to send emails and get to know those women.

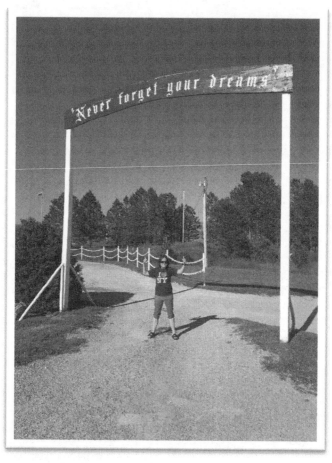

(Me standing outside Crazy Horse Memorial in the Black Hills of South Dakota. July 2018)

CHAPTER 14

My Dream to
Become an Author

Shortly after I was inspired to reach out to Ally, I wanted to reach out to a family friend, Kathy, in April 2018. I met her for the first time after I had graduated high school. Kathy and my mother used to work together at the Mountain Peace Shelter in Bailey, Colorado. I knew that Kathy had recently coauthored a book with one of her friends and published it. In April 2018, I was inspired to email her and ask if she would be willing to talk with me about her book and the process to publish it. Before I knew it, Kathy and I had set up a time to talk on the phone one weekend. I was excited to talk to her and see what I could learn.

Prior to talking with Kathy, I had already started writing my story. At the time, I had a piece that was a little over ten pages long. The day that Kathy and I talked on the phone, I gained an understanding of the next steps I should take with my writing. She was able to provide me with some valuable information and insight. At the end of the conversation, she told me to reach out again if I had any other questions. Talking with her made me believe that one day I would publish my writing. Kathy sent me numerous emails with information and even mailed me a copy of her book.

The conversation with Kathy motivated me to start doing some research on my own. On the day I talked with her, I researched publishing companies and how much it would cost to publish a book. Taking that step made me aware of how ready I was to share my story. Reaching out to Kathy helped me understand where to start the journey of publishing my story. Throughout our conversation, I learned a lot about the process of creating a book. I was so thankful that I had a family friend who could be a resource for me along the way.

Once I talked with Kathy, writing down my story became very easy. Talking to her gave me amazing motivation to write everything down. Before I knew it, the project that I had started with no intention of sharing had taken off. I was surprised at how quickly I was able to write. Ten pages became fifty in the blink of an eye. Each day, I wanted to write more. When I had any free time, I would sit with a cup of coffee in my office room and write. If I sat down at my desk to write, I could easily spend a couple of hours doing it. I was so motivated to write my story. The fact that I was writing something that could potentially be shared one day was extremely exciting. Something inside me told me that writing my story was meant to be.

Throughout the process of writing this book, a small group of people knew I was working on it. I was so excited about it that I couldn't keep it a secret. I remember one time being asked if I was certain that I wanted to share everything about my journey so publicly. Without hesitation, I answered, "Yes." As I continued writing my story, one thing that became clear was that I was ready to tell my story. I initially started this writing project strictly as a form of therapy for me. However, I quickly realized that my story was meant to be shared. It was once said that you should "be fearless in the pursuit of what sets your soul on fire." Writing my story and sharing it is what set my soul on fire. Once I knew that I was going to consider publishing this story, I constantly felt a positive adrenaline rush. That is how I knew I was doing the right thing, and that my soul was burning to let everything out. I then decided that I was not going to let fear or anything else stand in the way of sharing my story. Becoming a published writer quickly became a dream of mine. I encourage everyone to find what sets your souls on fire and pursue it. It is never too late to pursue your dreams. Don't let anything (especially fear) get in the way of chasing your dreams.

Getting this book published did not come without some challenges. As I did research, I realized that the process of publishing was more complex than I thought it would be. The idea of navigating through the process from manuscript to an actual book was a little overwhelming. There were times when my patience was tested. However, I learned that if you have a dream, you can find a way to make it happen. When my patience was tested, I wouldn't let myself get discouraged. The dream of sharing my story was worth fighting for, and I refused to give up. As I read through Kathy and Barbara's book—*A Place for Me! Empowering Wisdom to Create an Amazing Life*—I found a quote, "There is a vitality, a life force, an energy, a quickening that is translated through you into action and because there is only one you in all time, this expression is unique. And if you block it, it will never exist through any other medium and will be lost (Mastroianni & Webster, 2015)."That quote instilled a lot of motivation in me. I knew that my story was unique and promised myself that I wouldn't let anything block or prevent me from sharing it. Always fight for your dreams because they are worth it.

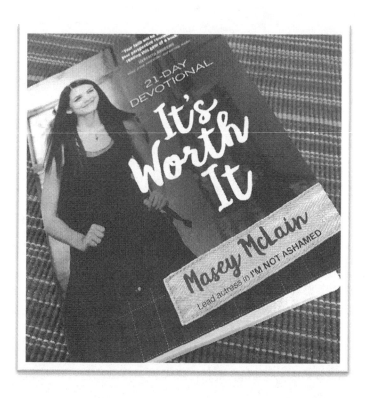

CHAPTER 15

Have Faith in Every Scene

I n May 2017, I read a book called *It's Worth It* by Masey McLain. It is one of the most powerful books I have ever read. If you haven't read it, I highly recommend it. It is a twenty-one day devotional that really puts things into perspective. Day two of the devotional compares life to a movie. The main point of the analogy is that not every scene of your life may make sense at the time it happens, but it is important. In a movie, every scene is important to the story and has a purpose. Just like a movie, every scene of your life has a specific purpose. The lesson from

Day two is that God creates our stories, and he is with us as we go through every scene of our lives. Comparing the scenes of your life to the scenes in a movie was one of the most powerful things I have ever read (McLain, 2017, pp. 14-17).

As I read *It's Worth It*, I reflected a lot on my life. Without a doubt, the scenes that took place in my life when I was learning about my diagnosis did not make sense to me at first. I was angry and did not know why my life was playing out that way. Frequently, I asked myself why my life had taken the turn it did. I asked myself why I had to live my life with a form of Turner syndrome. I wanted nothing more but to fast forward through those scenes. I now know that those scenes were important in my life. Were they difficult scenes? Yes. Were they emotional scenes? Yes, some of the most emotional I have faced. In the end though, those scenes have purpose in my life. Without those scenes, I definitely wouldn't be writing this book. I also don't think I would be the person I am today without those scenes. Having those scenes in my life made me a stronger person. When I am faced with difficult times, I just think about the things I have overcome in my life. Thinking about that helps me to get through challenging times.

I often reread the section of *It's Worth It* that compares our lives to scenes in a movie. Each time I read it, I think about how much truth there is to that analogy, and I am left in awe. Starting in December 2017, I found myself reading that section of the devotional frequently. My advice to anyone who comes to a scene in their lives that doesn't make sense is to know that it does have a purpose. Live in the moment and don't waste time dwelling on a scene to find the purpose. You might not find the purpose of a specific scene in your life right away, but you will find it. It took me twelve years to see the true purpose of certain scenes in my life. Have faith in every scene and live each one as it comes. If you are too caught up in trying to find the purpose of a specific scene, you never know what you will miss.

Reading *It's Worth It* inspired me to keep a gratitude journal. Every day, I write about what

I am thankful for. When I first started my gratitude journal, it didn't take me long to learn how powerful it is to reflect on the daily blessings of my life. Each day, I try to write at least two or three things (or about people) I am thankful for. Writing in my gratitude journal is something I look forward to every night. Journaling is part of my evening routine. If it hasn't been made obvious yet, I am a reflective person. I love taking time each day to reflect on how beautiful life is. Keeping a gratitude journal is something I would highly recommend to anyone. I believe showing gratitude each day can have such a powerful and positive impact on your life. I know that taking time in the evenings to write in my journal has helped me become an even better person. If journaling daily seems excessive, find a routine that works for you. I bet that if you commit to writing in a gratitude journal three to four times a week, you will notice a difference in yourself.

One thing I have learned since starting my gratitude journal is that there is something positive in each day to be thankful for. I will admit that there are days when it is difficult to write in my journal. On some days, I sit for a while asking myself, "What could I possibly be thankful for today?" When I have a rough day, it is hard for me to figure out what I am going to write. There are days that I start my gratitude journal with the line, "If I am being completely honest, today was a rough day, but I am thankful for…" Once I sit and reflect, I am able to come up with something. Sometimes, it is something small like being thankful for a hug that someone gave me in the hall at school to make me feel better. Reflecting on a day that may have been difficult forces me to change my perspective on it and find something positive no matter how small. When I write in my journal on days that were rough, I write about what happened, but I also write about the positives I found in the situation. Finding some of those positives help me get through challenging times. I'm grateful that I decided to start a gratitude journal.

Writing in my gratitude journal each day helped me to reflect on how far I had come in my journey with Turner syndrome. On April 9, 2018, I wrote, "I have seen the positive gains in myself since December 29, 2017. I have opened up to people about me having Turner syndrome. I have opened up doors of communication with my family (immediate and extended) about my condition. I have learned to empower myself (I will continue to work on this). I have gone to a doctor's appointment that made me anxious and reached out to other women who have Turner syndrome. Most importantly, I have strengthened my faith. I am incredibly thankful for all the positive gains I have made this year. Words cannot describe how it feels. I know I will continue to make positive gains. I feel like I am taking down barriers and taking down barriers feels amazing." Taking the time to reflect and write down that list made me realize how far I had come. It was an incredible feeling to think about it.

I mentioned that one of the positive gains I noticed in myself was strengthened faith. From December 2017 to March 2018, I definitely developed (and continue to develop) stronger faith. Many times, I turned to prayer during those four months. I prayed frequently for strength, courage, and guidance along the journey. I tried to devote time for prayer at least once a day. Through prayer, I could feel my faith strengthening. Praying had such a calming effect on me. I could not be happier that through everything, I've developed stronger faith. My faith definitely helped me get through the challenging times I faced. I believe that my prayers for strength, courage, and guidance were answered in many ways. Within four months, I was guided (and had the strength) to tell certain people about me having Turner syndrome, which provided me with an incredible support system. Throughout those four months, I also learned how much strength I have within myself. I'll forever be thankful that I came to a point in my life where I could strengthen my faith and truly learn the power of prayer.

Easter 2018, which happened to be April Fool's Day, my mom convinced me to go to Flatirons Community Church with her for the first time. She had been to a couple of church services at Flatirons on previous Sundays and really enjoyed them. On that Easter morning, I decided to give Flatirons a try after my mom explained it would be different from the Catholic Church service I grew up attending. I was intrigued and wanted to see for myself why my mom liked this particular church. From the first time I attended Flatirons, I was hooked. It was definitely different from the church service I was used to, but that is what I loved about it. Until I went to Flatirons, I had never been to a church service that made me reflect and think so much. My mom and I started going to services at Flatirons every Sunday. By going to church, I realized again how far I have come on my journey and how much stronger my faith is. Church was another place where I could reflect on my life journey and remind myself to have faith in every scene.

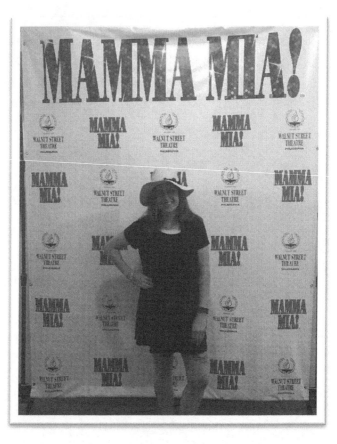

(Attending Mamma Mia! the musical in Philadelphia, Pennsylvania-July 2018)

CHAPTER 16

Summer 2018

On May 25, 2018, I officially ended my sixth year of teaching at Deer Creek Elementary. As I walked out of the school on that day, it was hard for me to believe I had already been a teacher for that long. As I reflected on the past six years, I would not have changed a single minute of them. Deer Creek Elementary was like a second home to me. In six years, I had created so many wonderful memories at the school. I felt like I was meant to be at Deer Creek and looked forward to continuing my journey as a teacher there.

As I started summer break, I knew I would have to get some medical tests done per my specialist's recommendation. When I met with the specialist over my spring break in March 2018, she recommended that I get an audiology test and cardiac MRI done. Both tests were recommended as precautionary measures. My specialist wanted the tests done because women with Turner syndrome can have hearing and heart problems. Even though I had previously gone through some medical tests for my heart and ears, it was explained I was at a point where everything should be checked again. Prior to summer break, I set up the appointments for both those tests. I found out both tests would be completed at the outpatient facility of the University Hospital in Aurora, Colorado.

Thinking about the medical tests definitely brought on some anxiety. I was most anxious about the MRI. Previously, my heart tests where EKGs not MRIs. I had never had an MRI in my life. Not knowing exactly what to expect is what made me nervous. I was nervous about being in the MRI machine. I was also worried about being claustrophobic; the possibility of them using dye for part of the test, and the amount of time the test could take. Leading up to the appointment for the MRI, my mind was racing as I thought about what it would entail.

One thing that became clear to me during the summer of 2018 was that I had learned some good coping strategies to help me work through anxiety. When I became anxious, I immediately would stop what I was doing and do something for myself. Often, I would put on my favorite spiritual song and pray. Sometimes, I would get my journal and write. Doing one of those things really helped me to calm down. During those moments, I realized that I had learned to handle my anxiety in a better way. I could see the growth within myself.

The first appointment that I had was for the audiology test. Overall, that appointment went really well. Once the testing started, it was done quickly. I left that appointment knowing my hearing was within normal limits. It was a relief for me to know that there weren't any red flags from that test. I was glad to have checked that appointment off my list. As I walked out to my car, I turned my focus to the MRI appointment. I was eight days away from returning to the same building for that procedure.

As I mentioned previously, the MRI appointment was making me the most anxious. When I scheduled that appointment, I realized it would be best for me to take someone with me. Once I decided that I wanted to take someone to the appointment, I immediately knew who that person would be. Terri was the person that I asked to come with me for support. As the appointment date approached, I talked with her on the phone a couple of times when I felt anxious about everything. I knew that she would be able to keep me calm and help me through the actual appointment.

On the day of the MRI appointment, I woke up thankful that I was going to have Terri with me. I felt anxious but was able to work through it pretty well. I spent the morning going for a walk around my neighborhood and praying. Both those things helped prepare me for the day. Before I knew it, it was time for me to go and meet Terri, so we could head to the appointment. We spent the entire car ride talking about numerous topics. Talking with her on the way to the appointment helped to keep me calm. My anxiety hit me during the car ride, but it was good to have Terri to talk to. I know I would not have been able to drive myself to that appointment.

When we arrived at the outpatient facility, I could feel my heart starting to race. I immediately felt nauseous and did not want to leave the car. Terri and I slowly made our way to the entrance of the building. After arriving at the radiology department within the building, everything seemed to go pretty fast. I was given a short form to fill out and then was called by one of the nurses. Terri came to support me as I was prepared for the procedure.

The first thing I had to do was change into some stylish hospital clothes. The nurse handed me some scrub pants and a hospital gown to change into. She then explained that after I was changed, I would go to another area where they'd start my IV. Hearing the word IV immediately made me very anxious. Prior to the appointment, I knew I would possibly need an IV for the test, so that they could inject dye, but that didn't make it any easier. Needles have always terrified me. Terri helped me calm down, and I went into the locker room to change my clothes.

After I was properly clothed for the procedure, I was not looking forward to the next steps. Terri walked with me to the area where they would start my IV. She knew I was most anxious about that part of the procedure. As the nurse prepared to start my IV, I got extremely nervous. Both Terri and the nurse told me not to look at what was going on. However, that was so much easier said than done. Terri was amazing through the whole process of getting my IV started. I was able to handle it the way I did because of her. Overall, the process of putting in the IV was quick. When it was over, I was so glad that it was done. The next step was going to the MRI machine for the actual test.

Terri couldn't accompany me into the room with the MRI machine, but she stayed with me until that point. Upon arriving at the procedure room, a doctor and nurse explained what was going to happen in detail. I was told that I would be in the MRI machine for an hour and half at least. It also was explained that I would be asked to hold my breath frequently throughout the procedure. After all of that was explained, it was time to get started. The doctors hooked me up to some heart monitors, covered me with some blankets, and then I was moved into the MRI machine.

Less than two hours later, I was done with the test. As I came out of the MRI machine, I felt exhausted. It doesn't seem like getting an MRI could be exhausting, but I felt like I could take a nap. Throughout the entire test, I was asked to hold my breath for varying periods. Having to hold my breath so much was tiring. Before I left the room, I was told I handled everything well, and that the images looked great. Hearing that made me feel like the process I had just been through was worth it. As I walked back to the locker room to change my clothes, I was relieved that everything was done.

Overall, I would say that my appointment went well. It wasn't exactly what I expected, but I felt

I handled it pretty well. There is no doubt in my mind that I handled it well because I had Terri with me. I am so thankful that I asked her to come to the appointment. As we drove back home from the appointment, I reflected once more about how far I had come since December 2017. I was at a place in my life where I had incredible people like Terri supporting me along the journey. I knew that the past five to six months wouldn't have been the same without their support. I could not have been happier that I had Terri to support me through everything that day.

Within a few days after the MRI appointment, I received an email stating that the results from the procedure were available to view online. Immediately, I followed the links within the email and logged into my account, so I could see the report. When I opened the procedure results, the first thing I saw was a note from the doctor. The note explained that the results of the MRI were excellent news. As I read all the information, I learned that everything from the procedure looked good, and that there were no major concerns. After reading everything, I scrolled up to see the note from the doctor again. Once more, I saw the words "excellent news." Seeing those words made me incredibly grateful and happy. I was happy that the test was over and overcome with gratitude for the good results.

Summer 2018 also presented an exciting opportunity for me. In June 2018, for the first time, I met another woman around my age who has Mosaic Turner syndrome. Back in March 2018, when I spoke with Marybel (the founder of Turner Syndrome Colorado), she offered to connect me with Nikki another woman with Turner syndrome. Shortly after that, Nikki and I started texting back and forth. With our work schedules, it was a little difficult for us to meet while I was still teaching. We remained in contact through text messages and agreed to meet once I was on summer break. On June 13, 2018, we went to lunch and met for the first time.

I don't think I'll ever be able to put to words what it felt like to meet Nikki for the first time. It was a surreal experience. I never thought I would meet another woman with Turner syndrome. Honestly, I was a little nervous as I walked into the restaurant to meet her that day. Once we got through the initial introductions, everything was fine though. It was great to meet Nikki and talk. She was such a sweet person. We talked about Turner syndrome and shared some of our stories. We also spent time talking about our careers, interests, and so much more. At the end of the day, I was extremely thankful that I had finally met Nikki. It made me very excited to have a new friendship, and I was looking forward to meeting with her again. I officially could say that I had met someone with Tuner syndrome and that in itself made me extremely happy.

Shortly after I met Nikki, I started teaching a summer school program for students in elementary through high school. I spent a week taking the students on various field trips within the community to do some project-based learning. That week is something I look forward to each summer. There is something so powerful about watching students learn through experiences outside the classroom. When that week was over, I knew I needed to get blood work done. That was the last thing on the list my specialist and I had created at our appointment in March 2018.

The Monday after the first week of summer school, I woke up and decided that I was going to get the blood work done. Of course, I was anxious because I knew it was going to involve a needle. However, I was determined to get it over with. I considered calling someone to go with me but knew that it was pretty last minute. Upon reflecting, I realized that if I had made it through the cardiac MRI, I could certainly do blood work. I kept telling myself that the blood work would be really easy compared to the MRI. Within fifteen to twenty minutes, I was in my car and driving towards Conifer for the blood work.

When I arrived at the laboratory for the blood work, I was surprisingly not as anxious as I thought I was going to be. I walked in and handed the nurse paperwork from my specialist with the orders for the test to be done. She took me back into a room and quickly got everything ready. Once everything was ready, she instructed me to sit down in the chair. I looked at the chair and then at her. Sitting in the chair was the last thing I wanted to do. When I looked at the nurse, she just smiled at me and said, "You can do it." I hesitated, but I sat down and within a couple of minutes, everything was done. I didn't even shed a single tear.☺ As I walked back to my car that day, I was shocked that I had just done blood work by myself. I never thought I would see the day that I would handle that test without someone there for support. I thought back to when I was sixteen when getting blood work drawn was a battle for everyone involved. Getting through blood work by myself that day was another moment where I could see the growth within myself, and it felt great.

Within four days, I talked with a nurse about the results of the blood work. She went over the results with me on the phone. As she looked everything over, she explained that they had done three different tests. She then stated that at first glance, everything looked within normal limits. When she said that, I'll admit that I did a happy dance. June 2018 had been a busy month for me with doctor's appointments. Talking with the nurse about the blood work results provided good closure to that month. When I hung up the phone, I officially had completed all the tests needed and had been given the results of each procedure. To know that everything was done (and that the results were all good) was a tremendous relief. On that particular day, I reflected on how far I had come on my journey with Turner syndrome and was awestruck once again. Within a period of six months, so much had happened in my life. I had come so far and was overcome with gratitude.

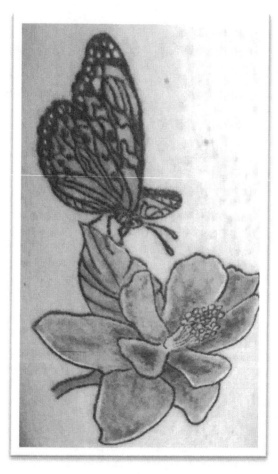

(Tattoo done by Charles Downey at Celebrity Tattoo in Lakewood, Colorado)

CHAPTER 17

Advice from a Butterfly

Looking back at the journey I have been on since sixteen, I realized that I essentially was living a secret for twelve years. I didn't intend to do that or necessarily want that. It is just what happened. I failed to realize I had been living a secret until I was twenty-eight. When I was sixteen, and I found out about my diagnosis, I believe I handled that situation the best way I could have. At sixteen, I decided that I was going to accept the fact that I have Turner syndrome and not let it dictate my life. At that time, I believed I had the choice to either accept it or go down a road where my emotions controlled me. I didn't want to let my diagnosis turn me into a completely different person. If I had let Turner syndrome define me, I know I would not be the person I am today. While I believe I accepted my diagnosis at the age of sixteen, I know that I never fully embraced it at that time. For years, Turner syndrome was something I avoided bringing up in conversation at all costs. It wasn't that I was ashamed of it, but I just didn't like to talk about it with anyone. Even though I accepted the fact that I have Turner syndrome, I had to learn how to embrace the diagnosis and let it be a part of me. At the age of twenty-eight, I learned to embrace my diagnosis completely and stopped living with it in secret.

My advice to anyone going through a similar experience is to just embrace everything. If there is something you have been holding back (for whatever reason), don't just accept it, embrace it. Along our life's journey, it's so easy to put up barriers. Never allow the weight of barriers to hold you down. It is so invigorating to embrace something that is a part of you and your life. As you have seen in my journey, so many positive things have come from embracing the fact that I have Turner syndrome. I talk with others openly about it now. I have found the strength within me to empower myself. I have built an incredible support system of amazing people, and I was inspired to write my story. Those are just a few of the positive things that have happened in my life. When I realized that I had finally embraced everything with my diagnosis, I felt like the weight of the world had lifted off my shoulders. I felt like I was free. Was the journey to get to that place in life challenging? I won't lie and say it was easy. It was difficult, but the rewards have outweighed the challenging times. I found that once I had taken down one barrier, the rest were easier to take down. Also, I learned that after you take down that first barrier, the adrenaline rush makes you want to keep taking them down.

In March 2018, I discovered a quote that really resonated with me. The quote by Alex Elle was, "Surround yourself with people who add value to your life. Who challenge you to be greater than you were yesterday. Who sprinkle magic into your existence just like you do theirs. Life isn't meant to be done alone. Find your tribe and journey freely and loyally together." Another piece of advice I have for anyone is to find your tribe. Find your tribe and let them in on your life's journey. One important lesson I learned at the age of twenty-eight was that your tribe would help you through anything! Letting more people in on my journey added to the tribe I have surrounding me. My tribe of amazing and supportive people got me through some difficult times, and I couldn't imagine my life without them. Embrace the people you are fortunate enough to have in your tribe. As the quote says, life is not meant to be done alone. Don't let anything prevent you from letting people in on your journey. When you're surrounded by people who bring out the best in you, the journey of life is a lot smoother. In 2018, I not only added members to my tribe, I realized just how blessed I was to have them in my life.

One more essential piece of advice I have for everyone is to take care of yourself. Don't forget to invest time in self-care. Starting in December 2017, I put a lot of effort into keeping up with the self-care routine I developed. Each day after school, I spent time doing things that I enjoyed and made me feel good. If the weather was nice, I'd go for a walk around my neighborhood. In addition, I would spend time reading for fun and writing in my gratitude journal. Each week, I also attended a yoga class. I found that all of those things really helped me relax and unwind after a day at school. When I forced myself to do self-care each day, I quickly discovered how important it was. There are days when it is difficult to take the time to do something for myself. Sometimes, I come home and think of a billion other things I need to do around the house or even for work. Following through with self-care makes a world of difference. If I don't keep up with my self-care, I can tell a difference in myself. I don't feel as relaxed or calm. I am still learning to stick to a self-care routine, but I can't stress how important it is. I would advise everyone to make the time to do something for yourself daily no matter what is going on. You will notice a difference in your overall well-being if you commit to self-care. The year 2018 has definitely taught me a lot about taking care of myself.

On December 31, 2017, as I watched the clock strike midnight and signal the start of a new year, I had no idea what was in store for me. I had no idea that 2018 was going to start with some challenges but continue with some amazing personal growth for me. In my wildest dreams, I never imagined that I'd get myself to a point in my life where I was motivated and inspired to tell my story. The year definitely brought some positive life changes for me, and I could not be happier that it happened. After years of knowing about my diagnosis, I'm finally revealing my true self. It feels incredible to let go of the barriers that were weighing me down.

Even though I vowed that Turner syndrome would not change the person I am, it has changed me throughout the years. Everything I have been through on my journey has turned me into a better person. Today, I am a person who holds nothing back. I have transformed into someone who welcomes being a Turner syndrome Butterfly. Gone are the days when I did everything in my power to avoid talking about my condition. The fact that I have Turner syndrome is something I will openly talk about with no hesitation. It's no longer private information. Without a doubt, I have grown into a stronger person through my life experiences. Starting in 2018, I was able to see many positive changes within myself. It is such a spectacular feeling to be able to reflect on life events and know that you have become a stronger person. I'm overcome with happiness when I think about how far I've come since I was sixteen.

When I initially found out about my diagnosis, I had no idea what kind of journey I was about to embark on. To be honest, I saw it as a journey that couldn't possibly be positive in any way. I didn't see anything good happening as a result of my diagnosis. The journey has had challenges, but I never envisioned how rewarding it would be. I'm learning that even though a journey may seem extremely negative at first, it can lead to some incredible rewards.

As I mentioned previously, I wrote this book hoping that it would help at least one person going through something similar. One day, as I was doing some research on Turner syndrome, I came across a quote about a butterfly. The quote was, "Perhaps the butterfly is proof that you can go through a great deal of darkness yet become something beautiful." I felt like that quote perfectly summed up my life's journey so far. Without a doubt, there are moments in my life that have been dark. However, I realized that 2018 was about making something beautiful out of those dark moments. It took me twelve years, but I felt like I had finally come out of my cocoon and become a butterfly. Life is definitely what you make it, and I am going to focus on making every moment truly beautiful. Each of us has the power to do that. You can overcome darkness and make it beautiful.

I never envisioned that, at twenty-eight, my life's journey would take the direction it did. If you asked me about talking to other women who have my condition, openly talking to people in my life about my diagnosis, or even writing a book at sixteen, I probably would have laughed. At that time, I didn't think I'd ever get to a point in life where those things were possible. In the Bible, Jeremiah 29:11-13 states, "For I know the plans I have for you, declares the Lord. Plans to prosper you, and not to harm you, plans to give you hope and future." In 2018, the direction my journey took showed me it was within my plan to share this story. Within a period of four months, so many positive gains happened in my life. I believe those positive gains occurred for a reason and really motivated me to tell my story. Once I felt it was within my plan to share this story, I completely embraced it and got to work. I've always been someone who loves helping others, and I'm hopeful that sharing this story has done just that.

Works Cited

Flippen Group. (2015). *Capturing Kids' Hearts Participant Manual*. Flippen Group

Mastroianni, K., & Webster, B. K. (2015). *A Place for Me! Empowering Wisdom to Create an Amazing Life*. Create Peace Publishing, LLC.

McLain, M. (2017). *It's Worth It*. BroadStreet Publishing.

Made in the USA
Columbia, SC
12 October 2020